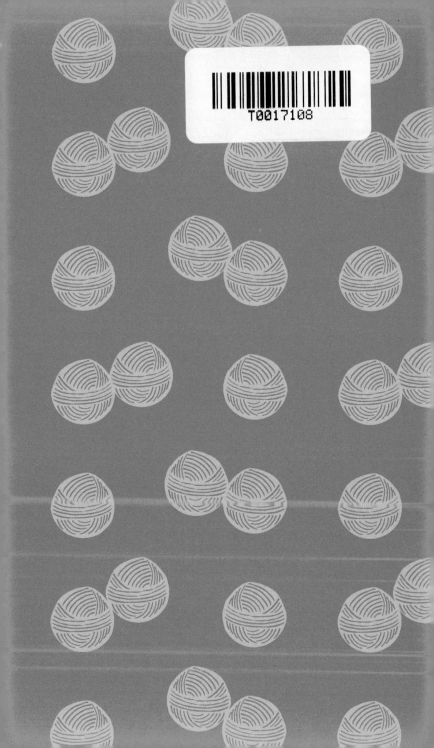

T0017108

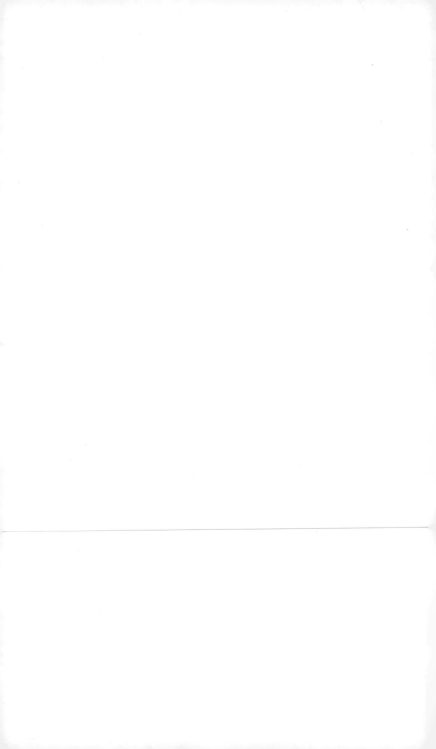

'Rachael Matthews is a true original,
a pioneer of the "new wave" of sociable,
expressive and fun knitting that emerged at the
turn of the millennium. This book celebrates
the practice of hand knitting as a meditative,
enlightening and mindful journey through
life, one that many can benefit from.'

SANDY BLACK
PROFESSOR OF FASHION AND TEXTILE DESIGN AND TECHNOLOGY,
LONDON COLLEGE OF FASHION

'I have been researching the meditative,
creative and social benefits of knitting since 2005.
This book adds significantly to the conversation
and in so doing gives knitting yet another
dimension to observe and explore.'

BETSAN CORKHILL
FOUNDER OF WWW.STITCHLINKS.COM

'This book is a delightful love letter to knitting,
and all the many beneficial things that come with
it. Rachael perfectly captures the home that the
craft gives us and helps deepen the understanding
of how we fell in love with it so hard and fast.'

BETSY GREER
EDITOR OF 'CRAFTIVISM: THE ART OF CRAFT AND ACTIVISM'

Mindfulness
in Knitting

Meditations on Craft & Calm

Rachael Matthews

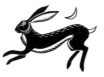

Leaping Hare Press

Quarto

First published in hardback in the UK in 2016.

This hardback edition first published in 2023 by Leaping Hare Press,
an imprint of The Quarto Group.
One Triptych Place
London, SE1 9SH
United Kingdom
T (0)20 7700 6700
www.Quarto.com

ISBN 978-0-7112-8821-8
Ebook ISBN 978-0-7112-8822-5
Audiobook ISBN 978-0-7112-8871-3

10 9 8 7 6 5 4 3 2 1

Design by Ginny Zeal

Printed in China

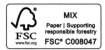

CONTENTS

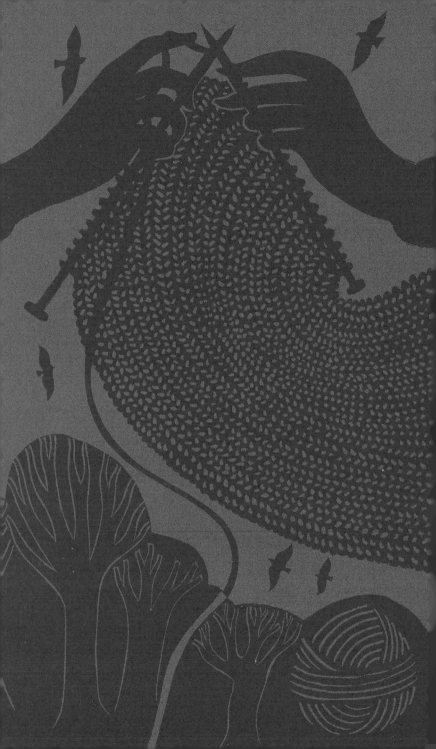

INTRODUCTION

*From the origins of society's natural evolution,
two ancient cultures have emerged, guiding the way
for our heads, hearts and hands. One of these cultures
is knitting, or to be more descriptive, the addictive
habit of forming a soft textile with your hands. The
other culture is mindfulness, or, as I like to think of it,
a childlike love of hooking up with your inner being,
listening to the pattern of your breathing and
exploring the flow of intimate thoughts.*

WHY KNITTING & MINDFULNESS?

Knitting and mindfulness have worked together over millennia to guide us through our growth. The utterly absorbing process of creating textiles provides us with an informal meditation space while connecting us with a heritage we cherish and ultimately a universe we understand.

A S TIMES CHANGE, NEW GENERATIONS knit different things, think different things and fit both practices into different lifestyles. This generation's rapid fads, economic downfalls and rising capitalism have called for our indigenous skills to reassert themselves with a passion. We have found ourselves longing to engage with a tangible material and form it into an authentic and functional thing to be proud of. As a hotchpotch of unwanted news images, adverts and social networking gossip buzzes all around us, the truthful heart of humanity whispers to us, 'Hush! Make something happen yourself! There is plenty of time to sort your head out!' The simple life of mindful knitting co-ordinates our heads, hands and hearts, helping our thinking become wider, deeper, freer and ultimately more interesting and creative.

Knitting as Medicine

Mindfulness and knitting may have been working together for generations, but it is only recently that the potential of their collaboration as a cure for ills has been confirmed. Scientists have proved that the repetitive action of knitting relaxes us, helps us think positively and can even be a cure for pain. Simultaneously, health officials are recommending mindfulness as a cure for many physical and mental afflictions.

Mindful knitting is here to help us find a joyous sense of awareness, where enslavement to repetitive stress no longer affects us. Even while we are making things, it is so easy to let our minds use us, rather than us use our minds. Our aim with mindful knitting is to create a new, productive and endlessly loving repetition.

Developing a more sedate range of thoughts, we will start to ditch the daily nonsense we usually carry around in our heads. When the mind is churning over rubbish, those thoughts do not dictate who we are, yet they can be all too easy to believe. Letting this rubbish disappear into rows of stylish knitting is a highly sustainable road to self-improvement. With junk binned and a knitting project cast on, we will focus on feeling at one with life, enjoying the company of a time-honoured craft, and the ever-evolving world around us. On this road to enlightenment we will find

---

Life is short, art long, opportunity
fleeting, experiment perilous, judgement difficult.

HIPPOCRATES (c.460–c.370 BCE)
GREEK PHYSICIAN AND THE 'FATHER OF MEDICINE'

---

plenty of places from where true wisdom and culture come. Connecting to nature through ethically made yarns will give us a tactile base for meditation. Introducing our brains to interesting number patterns in stitches, we will be welcomed into the world of mathematics, becoming part of one whole universe with no beginning and no end.

ABOUT THIS BOOK

◆

This book is compiled from all the experiences and conversations I have had with creative people since I was shown the joy of making things. I adore books, and in particular books that aim to inspire thinking, so it has been a pleasure to write about what I have learned.

I AM WELL AWARE THAT A BOOK SUCH AS THIS can only be a helpful tool and not a source of real culture, which can only come from the soul. This book is not a creative power, but a conversation to add to those wise provisions of tools that nature has equipped us with. I want the book to be like a telescope or microscope, assisting the study of your creative life, revealing unimagined wonders.

For years I was told that being well-read made you a good conversationalist. I was not a great reader or writer, but for some reason every knit project gave me something new to say. I now realize that the real sources of knowledge are not just books, but life, experience, feeling, acting and making.

Knitting, and talking about knitting, educates me about life. I am pretty sure that if you are planning to read this book you are already an enlightened knitter, with your roots dug in the love of materials and your thinking soul yearning to produce beautiful things. As you continue to ride on this wisdom, my wish is that this book can help you reflect on what is happening in your hands, in yourself and all around you, hopefully echoing my simple investigations in your own unique way.

How to Observe

Knitting, like mindfulness, offers a great lesson in *how to observe*. When we learn to knit, we must look at the stitches and pattern very carefully. Keeping a sharp eye on what we are actually doing, we must try to relax at the same time, watching our hands create an even tension. It may sound strange, but in learning to knit it can be easy to forget that *we* are doing the knitting … *we* must be the ones in control!

The three words '*how to observe*' also guide us through our development of mindfulness. Concentrating on our breathing and deportment, we learn to monitor our thoughts while relaxing at the same time. Again, it is easy to forget that *we* are doing the thinking, and *we* must be in control of our thoughts.

Capture thoughts as they fly through the mind, count stitches as they fly through the fingers; both of these tallies can be kept in order. With a tidy head and functional knitting, we can find peace of mind and something more.

Curing Boredom

If you are interested in knitting, the likelihood is that you are not idle. Knitters tend to have no time for nonsense, or any stimulus that wastes time in dead-end titillation. Knitters rarely suffer from boredom. Having said that, we have all been relieved to knit through a boring situation.

My granny says that 'boredom' is dangerous because it can only be 'relieved', but not cured, by adding something. It is easy to smother boredom with unceasing activities, making it appear that we live life to the full, but does it actually relieve the boredom we are covering up? For me, knitting works as a cure for boredom, because it provides the space to ask how the boredom arrived in the first place. Once we have drifted off into our repetitive state, we can ask ourselves: is boredom a symptom of wanting to be someone else? To be somewhere else? Or is it simply about not accepting that we are really here? Answering these questions while actually making ourselves a knitted gift is certainly a cure. The more we practise the acceptance and joy of being in the here and now, with production going on in our hands, the less likely it is that we will ever experience boredom again.

Clothing Your Loved Ones Twice

My biggest appreciation in writing this book is evaluating how much mindful knitting exhibits 'double the work' on show. The touchable aspect, the knitting, is easy to talk about because it is there. The invisible aspect of mindfulness puts on a show in a heavenly, abstract way, which others perceive but perhaps cannot describe.

In looking for a quote to illustrate this special aspect of mindful knitting, my father directed me to this passage from Proverbs 31, from William Tyndale's 1534 translation of the Old Testament. In this piece of writing, a housewife ensures that her family are 'double clothed' when the winter's snow comes. By this she doesn't mean putting on extra layers or thermal vests, she means clothed by textiles and spiritual strength combined.

> *She perceived that her housewifery was profitable,*
> *And therefore did not put out her candle by night.*
> *She set her fingers to the spindle,*
> *And her hands caught hold on the distaff.*
> *She feared not lest the cold of snow should hurt her house,*
> *for all her household were double clothed.*

Many of us are used to other knitters admiring our intarsia, or colourwork, and then cheekily looking on the other side to see how messy our tram lines are, or rudely running a thumb over our seams to check the neatness of our kitchener stitches. Mindful knitting confidently takes our 'other side' to a deeper and more insightful place. Through all the mindful work we are able to accomplish while knitting, the other sides of ourselves become quietly ordered.

CHAPTER ONE

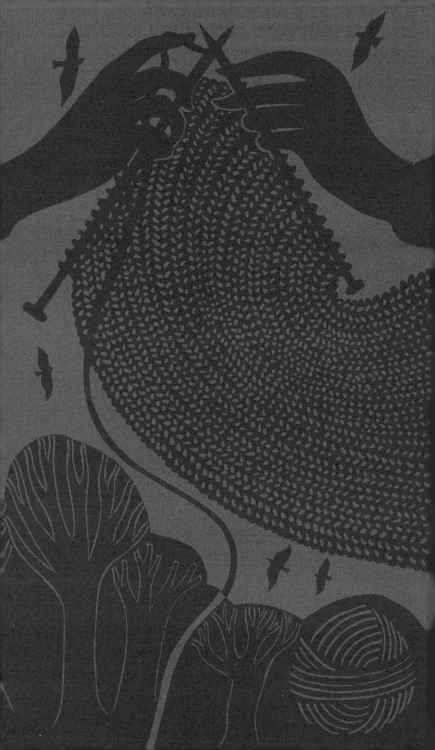

KNITTING, A LIFELONG STRUCTURE FOR LEARNING

*Your first knitting lesson qualifies you to
enter a rich dynasty of nimble-fingered, creative
people, who have made precious fabrics for thousands
of years. All your new associates have characteristics
a little bit like yours. That itch in your fingers that
inspired you to learn was possibly boosted by watching
someone else knitting, or feeling conscious of a family
tradition. Once knitting, you are not alone, and
through a lifetime you can develop an authentic
habit of meticulous work, made with head,
hand and heart.*

HOW WE LEARN

Practising meditation, we learn that some days we are ready to dive within, and other days we find it strenuous to resist distractions. Knitting has a similar training. With luck, our first lesson happens when we are calm and open to learning. Failure to learn because it's the wrong time is not the end. Try again later.

OLDER GENERATIONS SOMETIMES tell horror stories of learning to knit at school, producing embarrassing unidentifiable things and being put off the craft for life. Although the best time to learn to knit is about the age of seven or eight, when our motor skills are first developed, we don't always have an interest in learning to knit at that time. Then, later in life, inspiration strikes and adults are amazed to discover that the brain and muscles remember the stitches, and the work flows out as if their last lesson was yesterday.

Our 'domestic' craft is usually taught by a parent, grandparent or elder, or else we enrol in a knitting class. Finding the right way to learn can save a lot of struggles. The concept of knitting is amazingly simple in that every pattern is made up of only two stitches, one of which is the reverse of the other. Most people can learn the basic knit stitch in a focused hour. In practice, the full understanding of the mechanics, the responsibility of making stitches work for us, investigating how mistakes are corrected, learning to design what we want and finding the stamina to follow our projects through to the end are all lessons that are learned over time and by conquering challenges in the moment.

Being Present

The first step for a beginner is to find the right teacher, or if you want to pass on your skills, the right pupil. Chemistry between pupil and teacher is important. Elemental skills such as truthfully looking at what is happening, and thinking around what is really happening, are aided by both teacher and pupil being totally present and dealing with the looped thread of the now. Holding the work in a controlled way requires breath and clear messages to be sent to the fingers. Taking responsibility for the incorrect stitches we make, and being confident to correct the work, starts to make life's other problems easier to deal with. To an experienced knitter, these basic skills are obvious. Teachers are more likely to invent helpful and unpatronizing instructions when they arrive in the present. As the novice appears to wobble, we can also see progress; as nature joins up all the connections, the student needs to become a happy, flowing, knitting machine.

Adults who didn't learn a craft as a child can be shocked to find how unsteady their hands are in controlling the needles. Dexterity improves with every row, but the improvement needs to be noticed in order to be encouraged. Wobbly knitters sometimes forget to breathe or relax their shoulders, such is the fear of dropping a stitch. At every stage of learning knitting, the mature student can observe how the work feels, revealing much about the way they learn.

Learning or relearning to knit as an adult has the wonderful benefit of being more closely linked with mindfulness. As confidence grows and the rows increase, students notice that they are moving away from the 'to do' list. Adults have a deeper marvel at the way their fingers become a programmed machine, offering an engaged field within which to explore the mind.

Know Yourself

Whatever your preference for learning, whether it be an understanding teacher, vintage patterns and books handed down or found in charity shops, or instant YouTube tuition, it is important to recognize your learning style. Identifying the way you master the work helps you plan a comfortable path for your development, informing your teachers of your tendencies if necessary. Take note of your irritations with care. If the yarn is making you furious, take time out to study it in more depth, finding out why that particular yarn is not for you and how knitting could be easier in another colour. If the pattern appears to be lying to you, put your knitting down, sit quietly and find that inner confidence, which knows it can be on top of any instruction. Annoying mistakes that make you want to unravel hours of work and start again are actually little gifts in disguise. Place your knitting under a bright light in

EXERCISE

SKETCHING IDEAS

✳

The exercises throughout this book will enable you to develop a set of lifelong structures for learning. Start your first exercise by finding a new notebook and a pen that enhances your handwriting, feels beautiful in your hand and fuels you with a sense of adventure. Your notebook will be used to gather together thoughts about your life experiences, your ways of being and your knitting. Your abstract, psychogeographical adventures, where your thoughts wander while you are working, can also be documented here.

On your first page, start by drawing a wiggly line. This could be a decorative loopy tangle, or hold the kind of undulating kinks that yarn from an unravelled piece of knitting might have, bending up then down, up then down. Wiggle your way to the edge of the paper. (Wiggly lines are all knitting is when it comes down to it – loops working their way through loops.)

As your pen learns to behave like yarn, think about what you would like to learn from knitting. As the words come to you, work them into your wiggle drawing. Consider the bigger lessons in life, and characteristics you might need to fulfil your wildest ambitions. Let your thoughts build up a pattern on the paper. You do not have to stick to lines; draw your wiggle in rounds if you prefer. Decorate the lines themselves as if they were fancy yarn. Let the movement of the pen trigger thought after thought until you have filled the page.

a clear space and carefully trace the path of the misguided stitch until it is corrected. Ask someone to help you if necessary, and through fixing the error you will come upon a new fearlessness of future mishaps.

GROWING UP THROUGH KNITTING

❖

It is possible that the things we make deliver messages that other languages or actions cannot clearly express. Colour, texture and shaping express our identities in sublime and subtle ways. Sometimes these messages can inspire life-changing conversations, or reveal something memorable about ourselves.

I N THE SEPTEMBER OF MY TENTH YEAR, I was to start at a boarding school, 300 miles from home. My mother promised me that before I departed she would buy me a pattern and yarn for knitting my first garment. We went to our local wool shop, which had served our village since my mother was a child. Charmingly outmoded, the shop had orange cellophane on the windows to prevent fading, and an archive of knitting patterns from previous decades. The proprietor stood behind a mahogany and glass counter, sharp in a slim housecoat, with a perfect silver hairdo and fishnet stockings. I was excited to find a reasonably trendy pattern for a stripy off-the-shoulder number made with rows of lace stitches. To add to the excitement, I understood the pattern abbreviations. Taking my pattern to the counter, I was shown a selection of yarns that I was allowed to use with my pattern. I chose a navy blue double knit, and was presented with five hundred grams of fresh-smelling opportunity.

Apprehensive about the boarding school, the itch to cast on calmed my woes. Despite the yarn shop's provincial chic, my garment was going to be highly fashionable, and as good as any I had seen on television or in magazines. The garment would show people that I liked popular culture. I would prove myself an adult by knitting a whole garment. If I was still lonely I would enjoy the company of repeating navy blue lace.

Fitting In

I arrived at the school in a time when knitting had fallen off the curriculum many years before. Fellow boarders were taken aback to observe a hobby that only their grandmothers engaged in, and weren't quite sure what to make of me. Knitting suddenly felt like a lonely pursuit, as not even the teachers did it, and my mother wasn't there to congratulate me on my increasing rows. Feeling introverted and racing through the lace stripes, I finished the garment quite quickly. Surprisingly oversized, I styled it over a denim skirt of my aunt's, bunched up with an old belt of my dad's, parading my success with a mixture of empowered excitement and slight fear as to what people would think. The garment was disclosing hidden messages about who I was. Wearing the pullover helped me strike up conversations. The following year I was happy to find a knitting friend, and we were united with freedom of thought and deep friendship, bonded through the rhythmic duet of our needles.

The confusion my ten-year-old knitting self felt about fitting into the school community was probably no different from the feelings of the other children, with all their particular anguishes. What I failed to understand at that age was that when people fire a discerning look at your knitting, they are not attacking you, but merely expressing an interest in what you are doing. As well as seeing your product, they are observing your occupation of 'another' place, and to people who don't make things, that is most intriguing and memorable. Even if they think you are weird, it doesn't mean they don't like you. As an adult, I have visited teachers and pupils from school and they all remember my knitted efforts. My first jumper gave messages about the type of person I was growing into. I wanted the navy blue lace holes to express a certain type of sophistication and risqué fashion sense, which I was really too young to have. The pain of feeling out of place with an unusual hobby was replaced with self-assurance through modelling home-made clothing. Over many years, the sanctuary of the knitting process prepared me for resisting other people's preconceptions of who a knitter should be. I learned that it feels equally good to differentiate my style from others or conform to the norm, knitting replicas of things everyone else has.

A Spiritual Practice

The hidden spiritual culture that surrounded knitting was not tested like all the other lessons at school. The visible proof of finished garments was far more interesting to people than the thinking and feeling I must have engaged in through the process. To adults, my skills in producing knitwear were profitable, yet no one noticed the equally important value that the knitting had in keeping me in the moment and getting me through homesickness. Knitting through the now must have stopped me counting the days to the end of term. The conscious interest was of copying the attire of my favourite pop stars, yet my subconscious must have been aware of a humanizing effect, a secure space and an interest in spiritual affairs.

CREATIVE JOURNEYS THROUGH KNITTING

Like travelling, knitting has highs and lows. It's favoured for its portability and can be worked through long journeys and lack of adventure in equal measure. Whichever road you are travelling, your knitting offers a greater capacity for observing life as it swooshes by.

KNITTING IS A VEHICLE IN WHICH I TRAVEL. My knitted products are a diary 'on the road' of my life. The addictive nature of the craft grants a refreshed inner drive with each new project. Excited by our choice of pattern, we are fuelled with hope and intuition as to where we want to travel in our mind. Raring to go, with yarn in the bag, needles at the ready, the map is open to navigate our way to inner peace. Casting on is the key in the ignition of this creative journey. Revving up stitches and changing gear into a slower breath, we accelerate away from existing conventions of consumerism or hierarchies in society. We park up, switch the engine off and look at the view, loving our knitted cloth for what it is. As we get comfortable with knitting on the road, we start to imagine how our work could lead to revolution.

'Turn on, tune in, drop out' was a slogan used by the American psychologist and philosopher Timothy Leary in 1966 to address the original hippy generation who travelled huge distances across America to find enlightenment in a mass gathering. We could borrow Leary's slogan as a mantra for mindfulness in knitting, both for being on our own or within our community. The phrase encourages our journey of inward discovery and subsequent development of deep friendships, which can lead to social change.

Here's How We Do It

Turning on in knitting is easy; you literally just start. Turning on is a kick in the face of the procrastination monster. Don't worry about the list of things you need to do, as they can happen when you take a break after knitting a few rows. From the second you begin, time will manage itself differently. Don't worry too much about knitting the right thing, as you can always unravel the work if it goes wrong. Even on the days when you feel utterly useless or overwhelmed, the act of knitting proves that you are switched on, advantageous and in control. You are travelling along rows, moving forwards in the organization of your mind. As you let the stitches focus you on the moment, time stretches, and you cover great distances in yarn length. Turning on enables you to multitask by taking a trip in your mind and smothering yourself in gorgeous fabrics at the same time.

Tuning in happens once you have turned on. This is the actual 'trip'. As your working needles and breath anchor you into the present, the bustle of the outside world quietens and interesting ideas start to creep into your peripheral vision. Note these emotions and behaviours sincerely, as they are facts that can be mapped out and filed into your travel log.

The experience of turning on and tuning in has proved that you have dropped out of all the unnecessary pressure that society imposes upon you. You have become mindful of the worlds that are both within and without you, and your knitting is an action of pure individuality and strength. Cultivating thoughts and feelings sincerely through the journey of knitting and meditation leads us to much closer relationships with our fellow craftsmen. The harmony we feel when we find others who think and feel as we do gives us comfort and the freedom to host unclassified scenes. Knit your own flags of independence, and work within a peaceful structure, driving along on your chosen route with no sidetracking, hold-ups or tiredness.

LEARNING FROM THE PAST

❖

Knitting's usefulness and comfort is what destroyed most of its early history; we literally loved our knits to bits. Our ancestral craftsmen preserved the skills we use today, but often lost are the things they made and the stories of support they gave their communities.

THE VICTORIA AND ALBERT MUSEUM in London houses a pair of red Coptic socks, made in the fourth or fifth century in Roman Egypt. They have a divided toe, designed to be worn with sandals, and a contemporary feel. The socks appear to be knitted, but are actually naalbinded, the loops made with a sewing needle. Naalbinding is a forerunner to our two- or four-needled knitting, and I found it to be slow and intricate work when I attempted to copy the sock in three-ply, hand-spun yarn. The neat stitches, the brightness of the red and the fact that the exhibit survived at all, shows that these socks were made for, and by, someone very special.

I consider myself a skilled knitter, yet while trying to copy this ancient artefact, I realized my patience only borders on the requirements of an Ancient Egyptian Coptic sock 'knitter'. Pondering the foot's shape in this slow stitch, my composure of mind does as much work as my fingers. Settling down into the work, the mind teams up with the breath, enabling me to work for long periods of time, while the fingers, with their years of experience, manage the needle and thread.

The slowness of time-worn naalbinding is frustrating to begin with and I long to race ahead and bang out a similar sock on my four double-pointed knitting needles. Questions arise in my meditation. Is this a waste of time? Why am I doing this? What do I want to become by doing this? It is tempting to sidetrack with a cup of tea, but the breath keeps me working, and as the rows build up it dawns on me that my stitches are just another movement in nature's textile ecosystem, given to us to practise since our evolution. Whatever the outcome, people like us are programmed to do this kind of work.

Heads, Hands & Hearts

Whether we were naalbinding for a pharaoh, a Taulipang Indian of South America knitting on a knitting frame or a knitter from many of the cultures who pulled up loops with hooks (crochet), the knitting experience is as much about the occupation of mind as it is the working of fingers and the finished fabric. Knitting as we commonly know it, on two needles with knit and purl stitches, is a relatively new version of our familiar, non-woven fabric, and it is only in recent years that the effects of knitting have been proved by academics to be healing.

Those of us who have grown up with an ardent knitter in their tribe may have marvelled at the complex patterns that can be produced simultaneously with engaged conversation or gripping television programmes. The rhythmic flow of a knitter in the room is perpetual, smooth and sedative, just like a metronome or heartbeat. A knitter may systematically stop to whisper the counting of stitches, scribbling a small note on a scrap of paper. Occasionally knitters may halt in a fury, as a mistake is uncovered and a serious investigation is launched. As problems dissipate, the rows increase and, as if by magic, balls of yarn, needles, fingers and stretches of time will turn out fully functioning, finished things.

The diversity of knitted outcomes, made by many heads, hands and hearts with all of their peculiarities, temperaments and aspirations, are what make me love the culture of knitting. Textiles hint at the lives and loves of people. On showing your work to another knitter, it is possible that they won't be able to resist looking at the back of the work to try to find hidden clues as to your fettle.

Mindfulness Through Making

On completion, most knitted things will take on a life of their own and can become as normal to us as a second skin. Other things, not so wondrous, might be laughed at and never worn at all. Indeed, the biggest problem with knitting is that you can't try on a garment before you make it, and this is why the bygone times of knitting are embarrassed by so many disaster stories. Knitting is so often categorized as a lesser, common or domestic craft that it is easy to dismiss the skill, vision, patience and devotion with which all things, useful or not so useful, are made. Knitting is reasonably easy to learn, with books, teachers and now YouTube videos showing us a world of stitches, but the practice of mindfulness through making is rarely written about.

Someone, somewhere was probably knitting with us in mind in the months leading up to our birth. Tiny handmade garments are easy to forget about, yet can be passed down through families and communities for generations. As babies, oblivious to what we were wearing, we very quickly dribbled and kicked our way out of baby garments. Chewing the edges of various fabrics and contemplating their flavour, we became conscious of textiles in general, their weight, warmth, construction and our own personal taste. It is hard to remember when I first saw a piece of knitting and reflected on the enchanting idea that knitted things had been made for me by people that I knew. The possibility that they had been made while I was sleeping was even more exciting. As my dexterity developed around the age of seven, I was taught how to knit by my family friends. As the years progressed, I discovered how stitches work, and the characteristics of yarns. As the collection of my finished projects increased, my awareness of a 'knitting head space' also developed. As an adult, I find it helpful to see all my temperaments and peculiarities engaged at various stages of the project. Together, knitting and the meditative space it offers have provided me with a lifelong structure for learning.

Following Trends into the Future

Each era has its own reasons for knitting. Traditions are handed down from previous generations and we twist them from different angles, perhaps with a new sense of humour, or new material, into something that suits our life and time. Let's knit together all the contemporary issues we care about.

As previous generations hand down their skills to us, we can often observe their different mode for the craft. We want to inherit their skills and yet we don't always want to wear what they make, or knit the way they do. As we pass our skills on to our children, the same thing happens. Whatever our differing tastes, we have an opportunity to notice how knitting can be used in distinctive ways for each person, in their era, with their own uniquely developed culture. Questioning the difference in motives between generations of knitters is a key to finding out more about the lives of our fellow craftsman throughout the ages. Unearthing the textile histories of our family or our local area enables us to see how our own knitting experience is shaped by the culture of the past, and how we want to take those traditions forward.

Materials and social implications of knitting change with every decade, class and location. Ask your elders for their knitting stories. If your elders are no longer around, you could find their legacy in attics and drawers.

Hobby or Necessity?

My maternal great-grandmother was the knitter of our family. Some of her finished pieces remain, beautifully packed away, and I can sense from them that she was a glamourous lady who meticulously recreated contemporary fashions of the 1930s to 1950s. My great-grandmother had money, so her knitting was purely for pleasure. I can see from her attention to detail on the finishing that although she was proud of her creations, she might have been happy for them to be passed off as boutique-bought clothing. Living in the northern English countryside where only local wools were readily available, I was fascinated to find her stash of 'new' yarns like slinky viscose rayon, which at the time had to be ordered from as far away as London and Paris. For my great-grandmother, knitting must have been a hobby to fill long empty winter evenings, or afternoons of chat. A serious church-going lady, it is entirely possible that her knitting time was also prayer time, and I like to think I can see her peaceful thoughts filtering through her regular choice of dusty blues and purples.

Looking around the knitting history of my village, I find a different story to that of my great-grandmother. Country people are multitaskers, farming and tending to land, and sometimes working a second job as well; knitting at home would be a necessity for clothing the family and a way of earning extra 'pin money'. I can find evidence of the knitting in the local museum, but the mindfulness can only be imagined.

Studying these histories highlights my reasons for knitting. Glamorous slinky knits of the 1930s and the thrifty genius of knitting farmers are inspirational to me in equal proportion, and together taught me to question both the manufacture of clothes and the life benefits of learning a craft. Growing up in a consumerist society, my questions about where clothes come from are very different to those of my ancestors.

KNITTING AS THE HEARTH OF THE HOME

Contemporary lifestyles far remove us from the traditional portrait of the knitter, rocking in a fireside chair. Professionals now commute with their knitting and, once home, central heating offers the freedom to sit anywhere in the house. Yet knitters can continue to practise the magical, grounding principle of 'hearth'.

MANY ANCIENT CULTURES have a god of the hearth. Vesta, the Roman God of the hearth, gave us the English word 'focus', the Latin word for hearth. The concept of hearth can be created and tended through the focused action of knitting. The company of a knitter provides a similar vibe to the fireplace. Needles click where the fire would crackle. Where fuel waited to be burned, yarn waited to be knitted. As the fire heated the room, so the knitter provided warmth. The active knitter can focus on those gathered at home, and dwellers can feel focused by the non-verbal companionship

EXERCISE

PLACING OUR TALENTS IN HISTORY

✳

In finding ourselves, it can be interesting to think about the craft that resides in our DNA, inherited from our ancestors. Once we have considered these histories, it is fun to think about how we differ from them, what makes us unique to our cultural history.

Turn to a new page in your notebook. In the middle of the page, draw a little bubble (or whatever shape you are comfortable in) and put yourself in it.

Draw a horizontal line across the page, allowing the bubble to sit in the middle of the line. Below the line is the past, your cultural heritage; above the line is the future, the heritage you are yet to create. Probe into your family history and discover who made what and why. This is a great excuse to ring up long-lost distant relatives, bond with them over memories and tell them you are big into knitting! Note your findings below the line through a series of bubble diagrams. Feel your connection or disconnection from these stories and turn to the space above the line. In the last pages of your notebook you thought about the qualities you would like to develop through your knitting. Let these thoughts grow into active ideas, by imagining things you might make and reasons you might make them. Let these ideas be as wild as you like, all ideas are true, and some might manifest themselves in unexpected ways.

of the knitter. Conversations between loved ones buzz around our patterns of stitches. Conversations with ourselves are the deepest here. A solitary knitter ceases to feel isolated as they develop a deep meditation through their work.

Typically, the knitter's place is a comfortable chair with a large stash of yarn nearby. Tape measures and scraps of paper may lurk around making the place look busy. If the knitter is absent, the knitting might be draped over the arm of the chair or packed away into a bag. The gift we knitters leave behind is, of course, one of beautiful textiles, but alongside our material products we leave a subtle, unquantifiable atmosphere. Knitters take time to make beautiful and useful things, while considering the well-being of ourselves and those around us. Our non-knitting friends will rarely be able to identify the vibe we give, or the way we enrich the home.

Striking Sparks

As the tribe sees their knitter's projects start and finish, they experience an inventive phenomenon. Witnesses unconsciously learn how to appreciate beautiful things. Conscientious work becomes normalized. The self-respect of the knitter increases with every beautifully cast-off piece. Creating beautiful things not only moves great mountains within us, but it affects those who surround us in ways we may never fully discover. Making things can be exciting enough for a craftsman, but for a non-craftsman, the process looks like magic. A knitter starts with a glint of an idea and stokes it through to reality. Making truthful objects heightens others' beliefs in your abilities. Domestic textiles fill the home with other-worldliness, taste and a knowledge of how things are made. In an age of cheaply manufactured goods, the hearth of the knitter teaches an appreciation for handmade treasures and the art of focus.

With fire comes sparks. In over fifteen years of running textile workshops, I have witnessed constant sparkle, as knitting triggers enlightened thoughts in people. As enlightened thoughts empower us and ignite happenings, so the hearth becomes a place to reflect on our changes and experiences, kindling the next project, and so the cycle continues.

Enlightened Reflections

- How does knitting fit into your life now?
- What are the most enjoyable parts of your life?
- What are the most difficult parts of your life?
- How does knitting relate to your life?
- How does the physical aspect of knitting feel?
- How do your projects work out? Do you enjoy the finished product?
- How is your ability to work through life's problems while you are knitting?
- How has knitting changed your life?

CHAPTER TWO

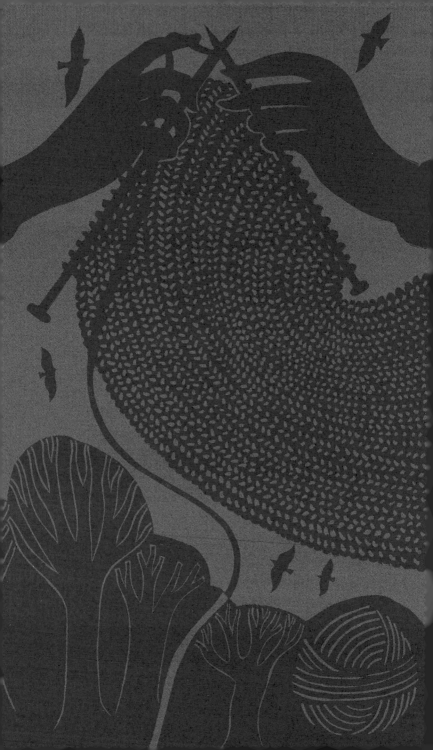

FINDING
OUR PLACE
THROUGH YARN

*In terms of human needs, textiles are of key
importance, alongside food, drink and shelter.
Our relationship to our second skin is profound,
yet we very rarely know exactly how and where our
trusted materials were made. Our attraction to certain
colours reflects our mood and this changes throughout
our lives. Our choices in textiles tell us much about
who we are and the culture that we live in. Noticing
the interdependence between colour, texture,
nature and human skills can deepen our
relationship to the entire universe.*

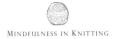
IDENTIFYING OURSELVES
WITH SPECIFIC YARNS

◆

Entering a yarn shop and facing a blast of the entire colour and texture spectrum can be overtly inspiring, blowing us away from our own unique and focused fashion. Intuition can be an exciting tool for choosing yarn, but this only works when our identification with it is truly founded.

MARKETING CAMPAIGNS SURROUND most of us, most of the time. Devised from deep studies of human emotion, they are designed to hook us, especially on days when we are feeling whimsical or slightly unbalanced. Deep within us, we each have an authentic taste that doesn't need marketing campaigns for inspiration. Our taste is structured around cherished memories and perceptions of how colours and textures make us feel. Considering how colours describe who we truly are helps us to become more mindful when shopping on the high street.

Forming relationships with certain kinds of yarn is deeply personal. We all have a favourite combination of foods, or an ear for certain rhythms in music. We might have developed these passions in childhood, or discovered new colour combinations on a holiday adventure or through falling in love with someone. Colour and texture help us connect our memories and can inspire conversations about our knowledge of the world.

Hardy Herdwicks

My most trusted yarn to knit with is also the one that I most complained about as a child: the itchy but beautiful Lake District Herdwick yarn. Herdwicks are thought to be a Viking sheep, and spend the year roaming the fells (mountains). We have many Herdwick references in our family, because legend has it we are descended from the Vikings who brought the sheep to England. My brother and I were reminded of this every time the itchy collars were pulled over our heads.

Herdwicks were championed by the famous children's author Beatrix Potter, who appreciated the way the wool repelled rain and mud when she was working her smallholding in the Lake District. When she moved there, the Herdwicks were under threat because local farms were being sold off and the farming community feared that their way of life would die out. Beatrix Potter bought up many of the threatened farms and continued to rent them to the farmers.

Potter was a Victorian feminist and rebel, taking charge of her business affairs and speaking her mind. The itchy yarn she championed reminds me of her defiant, strong nature. My grandfather was also defiant and strong in Herdwick when he survived the Second World War in the Arctic Circle wearing itchy long johns right next to his skin. When I knit with Herdwick wool, I feel heritage flowing through my fingers. I can't confirm if I am truly Viking, but I love playing my role of knitter and spinner in the next generation of Herdwick fans.

Gorgeous Greys ...

The tough little Herdwick sheep vary in colour but strike a stylish pose with their white socks, white faces and hard black stare. The lamb's wool is 'black' or rather dark brown, and as the sheep ages the fleece develops into blends of greys, with some parts turning white. Aesthetically, Herdwick has unusual effects. The blend of greys is never idle or listless, but rather alive with sparkling specks. I love knitting with it, because any colour or texture you put next to it is greatly enriched by its presence.

EXERCISE

A MUSEUM IN YOUR STASH

❋

Collect yarns that remind you of specific times of your life – magical times, or perhaps times you would like to forget but can't. Work up little samples of yarns and place them in your notebook. As you work the yarn, note down all the reactions you have to its touch. What do you remember? How does it feel? Have the feelings changed since you were young? How does the yarn represent the culture you came from? Does it have a place in your culture now?

Review your memories with an open mind, accepting that your creativity gives you the power to make change. Consider the relevance of these feelings to your life now. Use your knitting to rewrite your history, or tell a fictional story.

Do you need to knit a second sample? Has anything changed?

As I work the wool, I think of the numerous sheep hefted between drystone walls, which have a similar amalgamation of greys with their granite sparkles, lava tones and limestones. Drystone walls were lovingly built across the fells for miles, and as they age become richly coated in lichens of acid yellows, deep oranges and gentle chalky greens. The fresh atmosphere that lichens need to thrive is apparent in the vibrant saturation of their colour.

... and Acid Yellows

I didn't find the perfect companion yarns for my Herdwick until I visited the majestic Rocky Mountains in Colorado, USA. I was fortunate enough to stay with a friend in the remote mountain shanty town of Ward, where the Beat Poets had left their magic and many of the houses were self-built. In the middle of the town, at the back of the general store, was a little wool shop called 'Full Spectrum Fiber Arts'. Full spectrum it was, but only across the chromatic scale of acid yellows. Mary, the shop's owner, sold hand-dyed yarn sourced only from the surrounding nature. Ward is surrounded mostly by aspen trees, standing tall for miles with their knobby white trunks and wonderful leaves turning from green to bright yellow and eventually orange. Spending most of my holiday budget on the full range of rich beatnik yellows, I finally found the perfect friends for my Herdwick greys, a match made in heaven from two mountain ranges nearly five thousand miles apart.

Environmental Awareness in Yarn

Refining the manufacture of softness has happened over time. We are all privileged to wear softness near our skin, but this softness is such that it is easy to forget it is there. We do not treasure softness as we should. Taking softness for granted is ruining the planet.

As a child growing up in England, I was never fully aware of the problems cotton production had caused in the world. Cotton mills across the north of England had closed by the time I was born. Being a lover of folk music, I was aware of the terrible conditions that weavers had had to endure and their need for song to get them through their very long and uncomfortable days. When Richard Attenborough's remarkable film *Gandhi* came out, my eyes were opened to the enormity of how our greed for the Indians' soft cotton caused a revolution in India and ultimately lead to the downfall of the British Empire.

As I grew into blue jeans and investigated blues music, I learned about American cotton production and its reliance on slavery. The rhythmic a cappella songs relieved boredom, and improvising verses expressed frustrations and helped make connections with their fellow workers. I've loved my jeans so much (especially worn with a woolly jumper), but the comfort and ease they give me come at the end of a seemingly complex supply chain and a chequered political history.

A Sobering Experience

My understanding of the true cost of cotton came when I paid my first visit to a working cotton field on the edge of the remains of the Aral Sea in Uzbekistan, the second largest exporter of cotton in the world. A significant proportion of the Uzbek population work in the industry and the chemicals and water used to grow cotton are causing an environmental disaster. Since the 1960s, Soviet irrigation for cotton production has been fed off the rivers that feed the Aral Sea. Much of that water is lost through leakage or evaporation. The fish in the Aral Sea started dying in the 1970s as the waters began to recede. Fishing boats now lie stranded in the miles of dried-up seabed, like skeletons in the desert, while toxic chemicals, used to protect the cotton crops, are left as dust. Great winds blow these particles over the Uzbek population, who may go on to suffer with either tuberculosis or cancer as a result. Underinvestment and a shortage of agricultural machinery means that most of the cotton harvest is gathered by hand, often by children. Cotton farmers can be forced to sell their harvest to government-owned companies for a fraction of the market value. The state also controls much of what is needed to cultivate the crop, so often expenses outweigh income and, despite their labour, farmers can end up in spiralling debt. In May 2005, the cotton farmers attempted to hold a demonstration against these conditions, however government troops ferociously crushed the protest and many people were killed.

Countries in Europe buy a significant proportion of the cotton produced in Uzbekistan, dealing with corrupt politicians and businessmen in the process and helping enable this human and environmental disaster to continue.

White Gold

This was not the easiest information to take in on a holiday. The revulsion I felt at the world's greed for cotton was matched by the terrible tummy I had developed from eating greasy food fried in cotton oil – a substance that turns putrid in daylight and can only be digested by an immune stomach. My mind was blown as I witnessed this crazy system, while remembering the racks of t-shirts sold for one pound on the market back at home. The cotton buds themselves were so incredibly beautiful and the heap of cloudy white fluff, en masse, absolute heaven. Nature's gift of 'fluffy white soft stuff' is so incredibly special, and its new nickname of 'white gold' suits it well. The loss of respect for this plant and the way it grows was so different to the local history I was reading about and the monuments I was seeing on the tour. The stunning city of Samarkand located on the Silk Road, with its mosques, mausoleums and trading of treasures, would once have been busy with textile merchants trading silks from China. I was relieved to find there were still beautiful local fabrics for tourists to buy, adorned with highly skilled hand embroidery. The crafts were very much alive even many of the people weren't.

Homespun Cotton

On returning home I realized that I needed to improve my relationship with cotton, and understand its true value. I decided to start by sourcing some fibre, to discover its quality and find out how the yarn is made. Cotton will grow indoors in Britain but it can't handle our cold weather. My friend Annie, a textile expert, gave me some organic cotton fibre grown in America by Sally Fox. Top quality and ethically made, it also grows in three different natural colours, white, pale green and orangey cream.

At my spinning wheel, I found Sally's short cotton fibres challenging after the long, strong, sticky fibres of wool I was used to. Slowing the wheel, I eased the short fibres in much faster than usual, while little bits floated up into the atmosphere and sometimes up my nose. Wanting to mix the short fibres with a longer staple, I carded in some long recycled silk fibres, in shiny, bright multi colours, which conjured up a vision of many caravans of camels carrying their bundles of beautiful treasured fabric across Uzbekistan.

I needed to improve my relationship with cotton

My finished two-ply yarn was soft beyond belief, a solar halo of an iridescent rainbow cloud. I couldn't bring myself to knit with it as it held so much spirit just sitting in the skein. It remains completely functional as a bundle of bliss for resting my head on, while thinking about the flow of fresh water and fibres across the planet.

Gandhi's Charkha Wheel

Wanting to make a more durable cotton thread, I then set about trying to spin thin and tough just like Gandhi did. I purchased one of Gandhi's charkha wheels, which folds away into a cigar box. Gandhi designed this wheel as a tool for every household across India, encouraging the population to grow cotton in their gardens and spin yarn in their meditation time. Winding the handle and letting the fibres slip off my thumb, this was spinning on a minute scale, where tightness of spin gives a crisp and precise thread. As much as I loved spinning the cotton in my rainy London studio, I couldn't help wishing I was working in heat and sunshine, dressed in one precious homemade piece of cloth.

EXERCISE

PLACING YARNS ON THE MAP

✳

In this chapter I have described two of my deepest relationships with yarn. The first was an itchy fibre from rainy northern England and the second a soft fibre from far-off lands where the sun shines brightly. Your top two favourite yarns are likely to be quite different to mine. In this exercise, take time to consider which two yarns best describe your character. Engage with the yarn on a deeper level, finding out where it comes from and, if you can, arranging a visit to that place, either virtually or for real.

ITCHY VERSUS SOFT

In my wool shop, my customers often scanned the yarns and asked, 'Do you have anything soft?' The softest collections weren't soft enough. Nature's variety of textures can invoke many feelings and sensations. Let textures open our awareness to how the planet can ethically clothe us in a complex variety of softs.

THERE ARE OVER TWO HUNDRED BREEDS of sheep across the globe. Sheep have been bred over thousands of years to provide distinctive qualities of yarn, ranging from itchy durable to super-soft. Alpaca, a little South American camel, is now added to this list. It is top of the soft rating as it is lanolin free, making it hypoallergenic. Collecting rare breed yarns, I have learned that there should be as many words for 'soft' as there are Eskimo words for types of snow. Silky soft, spongy soft, floppy soft, solid soft, delicate soft, durable soft, soft when you are comfortable in your skin, soft when you are not comfortable in your skin.

The Lost Art of Wearing Wool

My experience of running a wool shop has prompted me to question whether our skins are becoming more sensitive to wools. Knitters often feel threatened by wool and struggle to find a natural, ethical fibre that is softer. I suspect that our skins were always sensitive to lanolin and the prickle of wools,

Hair Shirt

Thomas Becket, Archbishop of Canterbury from 1162 until his murder in 1170, is famous for his hair shirt, worn close to the skin to induce discomfort or pain as a sign of repentance and atonement. Other irritating features were added, such as wire or twigs. The fad for the itch still survives in religious ceremonies today, and although our itchiest wools could be a perfect punishment, I do not consider suffering to be necessary in our mindful consideration of yarn usage.

but we *are* forgetting how to build up our softer under-layers. Wearing two or three layers of clothing has become too hot now we are cocooned in central heating. When I teach textiles in the university, I have to dress for the central heating, wearing one thin under-layer and a lightweight top layer. On the days I wish to impress my students in a traditional Aran cable jumper or fuzzy Shetland Fair Isle, I tend to overheat.

Merino, one of the world's softest-to-the-skin fleeces, has become the popular wool of choice for its lightweight, soft, bobble-free nature. Mixed with overly produced cashmere, it is even more marketable. Checking the supply chain of your materials is significant as it can uncover stories of animal abuse. Alternatively, your purchase could be supporting a conscientious organic farm.

FINDING THE MAGIC IN COLOUR

Colours cannot be classed as good or bad, only as 'true'. Nature teaches us that the colour spectrum works in perfect harmony, and through playing with the placement of colours we find their affinity with each other. Mindfully noticing this reminds us how our own energies and emotions balance.

THE METEOROLOGICAL PHENOMENON that we call the rainbow sends shivers of delight straight through us as we happen upon it. With or without a deep understanding of physics, the purity of colour is always astonishing. A shaft of sunlight passed through a glass prism is equally enchanting. The rainbow is nature's presentation of colour in purest form.

Rainbows sit soundlessly, as they triumphantly display the colours that reside in the rest of nature. There may even be more colours that we cannot yet see. As light moves around, the colours around us darken, lighten and play wonderful games. The rainbow's translucent colours may fade, but for that short time they may beguile us into finding a more permanent luminosity elsewhere. The rainbow hints at colours that are hidden in flora and fauna, just waiting to be extracted as natural pigments. The rainbow is always beautiful and there is no colour within it that does not bring us a deep sense of wonder or contentment.

The colour spectrum works in perfect harmony

Emotion

Colour depends not only on the quality of light under which we see it, but also on the ability of our eyes to truthfully receive the colour. When we are unconscious in the present, or feeling low, we might not perceive the power of colour. When we are alert and feeling perceptive, the differentiation of colours deepens and exciting things start to happen. Colours dance, changing each other by their juxtapositions. Some colours radiate, while others withdraw into themselves.

Back at the wool stash, we can investigate the abstract quality of our emotions by carefully arranging yarns, letting them form relationships that hint at our mood. We do not need to clarify that mood intellectually, as the colour spectrum is not an intellectual scale. Find colour stories that satisfy different moods, take you out of your safety zone and evoke a sense of freedom.

Language

When I learned the colours of the rainbow as a child I recited the very English mnemonic 'Richard Of York Gave Battle In Vain', which helped me to remember the colours Red, Orange, Yellow, Green, Blue, Indigo and Violet. The names of these colours were only the beginning of a colour language. Running a wool shop, I often have fascinating conversations with knitters as they search out the perfect hue for their design. Look down the catalogue list of any yarn or paint company and you will notice references to sciences, arts and humanities written in the most creative ways.

Illustrating colour schemes with words requires us to become poets, trundling through the archives of our memories and sifting through the labyrinth of our emotions. Once we have conceived our colour story, we have a rare, personal tale to tell when someone asks us what we are knitting. My love of yarn from the mountains gives me a foundation to describe my childhood. The yarn provides me with a conversation opener, where my enshrined subject might not otherwise have been exposed.

In Pursuit of a Colour Buzz

This morning, I made my coffee and then started my hunt for a morning colour buzz. These appear when you least expect them. The first job on my list was to sort out my recycling bins. One can find endless colour inspiration in bins. From the colour chaos of today's bin emerged an urge to lie on a lounger on the edge of Italy's Lake Como with a dry Martini in one hand, wearing a large sun-hat and quite a daring new colour palette. The hard plastic green of my semi-skimmed milk bottle lid, placed next to the shiny gold wrapper of my partner's new battery charger, seemed very exciting. Both of these samples are synthetic, but when placed on a backing of crumpled brown envelope, they took on a more earthy, jewel-like presence. I loved the twist of the synthetic quality along with my memory of something ancient. I envisioned a loose-fitting dress, with matching sunhat, in natural brown linens with hints of green and gold rayon.

Studying rubbish is great for growing colour confidence. It is one short opportunity to find connections between the contents and investigate what is exciting at this moment. Meditating like this helps me to notice inklings of recognition in things, developing creative connections and learning new tricks to see things differently. It also brings a glamorous feel to a rather mundane job.

NOTICING INTERDEPENDENCE

The benefit of growing older is that we gather more skills, more knowledge of materials and the sublime wisdom of all the best craftsmen. Part of that wisdom is understanding our role in the universe. Respecting first principles, we embrace the world around us and give thanks for all we have learned.

I FIND HERDWICK A COMFORT TO KNIT with because I have learned enough about the wool to see myself as a small part of the supply chain, working the fibre from sheep to shoulder. I want to be part of a long tradition of people who have worked with this unusual fibre. James Rebanks wrote a beautiful account of his farming year in his book *The Shepherd's Life*. Learning about his early-rising, weather-enduring, tough, passionate and obstinate way of being has allowed me to feel even more connected to this wool, noting my interdependence on all aspects of the supply chain.

EXERCISE

TELL YOUR COLOUR STORY

✳

Arrange snippets of colours that inspire you on mood boards, in boxes or in sketchbooks. Share them with your friends and tell your story. Encourage them to do the same. Uncover colour responses through group discussion, as a way of getting to know your friends and their histories. Swap samples over a cup of tea. Perhaps your friends' memories and associations with colour will trigger your own memories or ease you into a colour scheme you had failed to identify. Next time you go to a yarn shop to start a new project, you will be much clearer about what you need.

Take the exercise deeper by focusing on the materials for a long time and letting them take you on a journey across the world or, if you'd prefer, forwards and backwards in time. Researching the cultures surrounding materials adds more depth of character to them or enhances your own personal identification with them. Release certain materials from their social stigma by seeing them in more worldly ways. Focus on the material and notice the images that pass through your mind. Studying your creations in this way will give your work a more truthful identity. The authenticity of your designs is multiplied when your relationship with the material has depth. We are the ones who make our materials come alive and in turn they comfort us.

Knitting a thick over-sock for wearing with a Wellington boot, I consider the entire process of making a garment. As I cast on the first round of rib, I feel a connection with the folk who pile on layers of clothes at 4am, to battle their way through miserable storms to see to the lambing of their ewes. Working up the rounds of stocking stitch, I remember the inquisitiveness of the sheep on the fells, staring at me as I hike on past. As I stripe my yarns I appreciate the sweating brow of the farmer as he shears fleece after fleece. As I correct mistaken stitches, I commemorate the cruel facts that sheep tails need docking, young rams castrating and a sheep's life isn't always as idyllic as it seems. As I divide stitches for the heel, I consider the generations of knitters who developed this technique and handed it down to me. As I cruise along the foot, I give thanks for the prolonged summer sunshine that enabled the farmers to make hay for the sheep's winter feeds. My garment finished, I wear respect for the farmers who declined the offer of a 'more sophisticated' life and advanced their family's farming dynasty. As I feel the snuggly soft warmth of my toes, I send respect to the sun-stroked cotton farmers, so far away from my cold northern European home.

The Five Dharmas

Contemplating the interdependence of things within our knitting practice can also bring us closer to the outside world. We depend on the producers of our yarn, and they in turn need us. We depend on our teachers, and once we have learned our craft, we love to pass it on. If we live in the city, we can knit ourselves a connection with the countryside. If we feel lonely, we can knit a dialogue with a world we would like to be part of. Contemplating the connection of things helps us to understand the interdependence of all aspects of ourselves. Our feelings, perceptions and physical awareness are all connected to each other. Buddhist teachings group the objects of the mind into five 'dharmas':

1. Bodily or physical forms
2. Feelings
3. Perceptions
4. Mental functionings
5. Consciousness

Knitting along with the dharmas helps us connect our being and our knitting to the (entire) universe.

Bodily or Physical Forms
Knitters often focus on bodies and physical forms in their work, contemplating existence by making comfortable layers to wear between the figure and the outside world. Knitwear can be designed as a way to blend in, or as a protection from the world around us. Through the making of garments, we often imagine ourselves or our loved ones wearing the piece and consider how they might feel. Our comprehension of

how the knitting could make us feel is based on the many images we have captured over the years. In contemplating these images and designing our projects, we might appreciate the designers of yarns who had a similar inspiration to our own. As designers, we may feel the presence of other cultures and times, tracing them back through history and carrying our ideas forward for future generations to enjoy.

Feelings

As we knit, feelings flow in and out of our minds. Some of these feelings come attached to a story, some can be classified as commonplace, whereas others are hard to explain or pin down. As we knit, we catch feelings, accept them and let them reside in the knitting. As we relate our feelings to the other dharmas, we see them as energy, passing through and informing us of the part we play in a much bigger picture.

Perception

Combining an understanding of natural materials, dexterity in crafts, awareness of physical forms and acceptance of inner feelings fuels our powers of perception. I'm always amazed at the ways ideas appear. Some grow gradually, emerging from somewhere deep, gathering energy as they come. Simple addition can form new concepts, as two ideas merge to shine a new light. Eureka moments ignite with a mind-blowing explosion, which is sparked by a mixture of understandings brewing in our knowledge. Perceiving the right gift to make for ourselves or a loved one needs us to contemplate physical forms and feelings, interacting with the universe.

Mental Functionings

As we become fluent in knitting, new mental functionings become multifunctional. Our skills are transferable. Our expertise is gained not through words, but through hands-on experience. This training becomes second nature, and we can use it as a foundation for other meditations. Our craft offers a space to extinguish unproductive thinking, relishing solitude and feeling comfortable with our place in the world. Our mental functionings at public knitting events are equally brilliant. Engaging in conversation while working stitches is very clever indeed!

Consciousness

The final dharma allows all the previous dharmas to be explored. Consciousness infiltrates all aspects of the mind and all the qualities of our knitting. If the world did not exist, we would have no reason to knit. The next time you finish let's say a hat, consider the existence of all things we consider 'the non-hat world': the places where the fibre was grown and the colours processed, the people who farmed the fibres and colours, the factories who turned the fibres and colours into yarn, the people who trade in the yarn and make our needles and the generations of craftsmen who taught us.

CHAPTER THREE

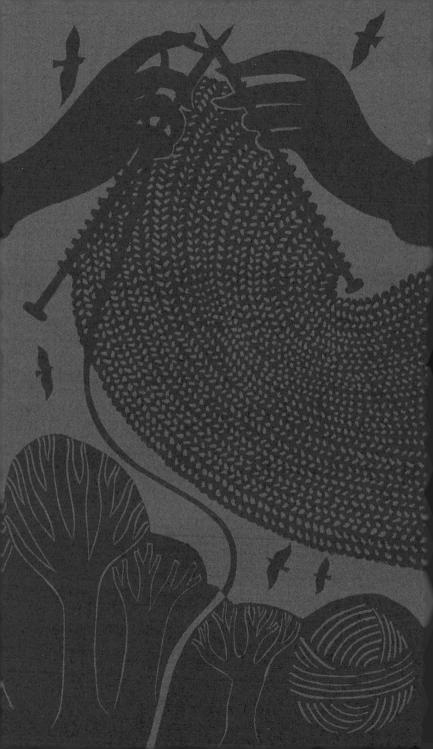

KNITTING
SACRED SPACES

*Deep within a knitter is a unique home.
Let us call this the 'sacred space'. A sacred space
is built around the heart of creativity; fortified by
experience, it grows to become a safe place for us to be,
make things and find our wisdom. Sacred space offers
us peaceful isolation to develop a craft, privacy to
evolve ideas and the mindfulness needed to follow our
inspiration through. Once we have learned the routes
to our sacred space, and some tricks to prolong
our stay there, we can visit it easily and
become productive and happy knitters.*

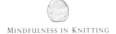

OPENING A SACRED SPACE

A 'messy' head can be liberated by the ritual of knitting mindfully. Our knitting ritual needs to be met with positive foresight, as we want to use it to reach our sacred space. Physical sacred spaces might ask you to remove your shoes, but entering into our sacred knitting space needs other preparations.

THE TERRITORY WE CREATE WHILE KNITTING is easy to take for granted. Knitters know their craft, which offers them a time to slow their rapid thoughts, but it is easy to switch off too much, get lost in our work and let the mind drift. Falling into our knitting is similar to the way we kick off our shoes and flop into our favourite armchair. Our hands remember how to knit, miraculously doing all the work and making it easy for us to cruise along in a lazy, semi-conscious state. Completing rows through a movie or gossiping with friends, we forget all about the here and now by escaping into other worlds. Measuring the knitting at the end of the day, we delight in the progress made while our minds were elsewhere. The escapism knitting provides, with its relief from boring situations or downtime with hours of daydream, is seductive because it is also productive. Awakening from the dream, we present ourselves with beautiful knitted gifts, knowing that the time spent away was reasonably well justified. If your work began with your mind in bad shape, it is possible to feel

EXERCISE

RESTARTING YOUR MINDFUL KNITTING PROGRAMME

✳

As you take up your needles, pause with a half-smile. Notice the lighting up of the face, the stirring of the heart and the calming of your mind. Take note of your breathing. Finding the rhythm of your breath, you are ready to engage with the rhythm of your needles. Working breath and stitches together, let the knitting guide you down to a place of calm. Measure your stitches with long breaths. Continue in this way until your fingers need a break, or you need to check the knitting pattern instructions. As you pause for a break, notice the work you have made since you entered the sacred space.

Take time to respond to the rows you have just worked. As you handle the material, remember your last knitting date. Answer these questions in your notebook: How does today's mood differ? Where do you want to go from here?

more relaxed by the time you put the needles down. Using a more mindful approach at the beginning of the session can help you find relaxation on a much deeper level. Let us ensure that a 'bad day' is transformed into a truly enlightened day through an extra structured practice.

Mindful knitting, once learned, is a companion for life and, like all great friends, it stimulates us and triggers enlightened thoughts. Cultivation of enlightened thoughts requires us to do some extra work. By our very nature, knitters love extra work! For our knitwear projects to become spiritually fruitful as well as fabulously stylish, we are obliged to switch on the right channels of the mind from the moment we cast on. Readying ourselves with a countdown to starting, we attempt to enter our sacred space exclusively, acting as a warden for sidetracking reveries.

Knitters as Computers

The hand-knitter could be credited as being the original portable prototype for the home computer. In the mid 1800s, Lord Byron's daughter Ada Lovelace was working with the inventor of the first computer, Charles Babbage. Lovelace recognized how the programming of the jacquard weaving loom could inform the first computer 'program'. While watching the threads of the loom engage as ups and downs, Lovelace grasped her concept of zeros and ones, programming patterns just like we knitters work guernsey designs in forwards knits and backwards purls. Ups, downs or forwards, backwards became holes and no holes before developing into zeros and ones. Our ability to create knitting patterns is as genius as the workings of a computer. We are able to work in extraordinary multitasking ways, talking and thinking at the same time as working complex patterns. Like any computer, we can break down and require maintenance and upgrades to keep us up to speed. From the moment we pick up the needles we start up, engaging in all we remember about making stitches. We are the machine. Our fingers are clever at

Knit Away Your Stories

A handmade piece of knitting with good tension and a spiritually enriched handmade piece of knitting with good tension, both following the same pattern, are likely to look the same. As we knit, we produce other, invisible works of great value. Take time to acknowledge this invisible work. Published knitting patterns do not normally provide meditation structures. Adding our own structures and rituals enhances your work time with a deeper source of personal creativity.

Feelings about the past and the future pass through our knitting constantly. Thoughts are facts that can be neatly filed away into the fabric, enabling the present to be less cluttered and free for more mindful knitting. Let your processed thoughts flow with the yarn into the knitting. As your rows build up, let your stories of the past and future leave the present, and find a suitable place to rest within the knitting. Note these thoughts in your notebook if it helps. As the stories are knitted away, notice the sentiment behind them and, with a clear head, continue to form useful, beautiful fabric. Woes will start to evaporate into your knitting rather than reside in your body. As you knit more rows, continue to demonstrate this simple filing system, until you feel you have fully entered your peaceful, sacred knitting space, and are free of any niggling fears.

knowing what to do, mechanically working the knits and purls and managing to count number patterns without our full attention. Sometimes when our computer brain is slow, it crashes or gets stuck. Like a machine, there are times when we need to shut down and restart.

If your mind wanders at the beginning of your knitting time, it is hard to rein in your thoughts while your fingers are racing on ahead without you. Start your knitting with a clear screen. Close all the other programs that shouldn't be in use, ensuring that you are working with your faculties in their most productive state. We could start our knitting session in the following way.

LISTENING TO THE BODY, OUR MACHINE

Academic studies prove that knitting can have a healing effect but taking psychological comfort from repetitive movements can cause physical strains. Responding to warnings from the body, we can do what we love without fear of injury if we live by Oscar Wilde's advice: 'Everything in moderation, including moderation.'

MOST KEEN KNITTERS WILL READILY ADMIT to being 'hooked'. A beneficial addiction, knitting can be taken with you everywhere, is relatively cheap and doesn't do any serious damage. Those suffering from harmful cravings can become the most productive knitters. If you weren't aware of an addictive personality before you started knitting, you might well discover a serious itch on completing your first successful project. The moreish process of producing stripes, intarsia or cable patterns can keep us working way beyond our body wishing to say goodnight.

Much of the practice of mindfulness is about reducing limitations. Narrow-minded circles of thought or excuses for not doing what we love gradually disappear through our creative meditation. Mindful knitters learn to relate their work to the entire universe, and beyond. Deep insights into ourselves and the world around us free us from any potential traps of misery. With all of these opportunities for positive stimulation, it is shocking to find that our posture can create annoying, miserable traps.

Check Your Mechanics

Preservation of our machine-like hands and arms is crucial to ensuring perpetual motion in our knitting. Evolution has ensured that our mechanics are perfectly designed, so long as we don't abuse them. I recently had an interesting conversation with two friends, a surgeon and a puppeteer, about warming up our fingers before we start work. My puppeteer friend explained how she warms up her fingers, hands and wrists before a performance. She likened it to the same ritual that pianists perform before walking on stage. My surgeon friend was amazed, as the sensitivity of his touch while he works is so important to him, and of course he has the ritual of washing his hands, but no one had ever suggested that he warm up his fingers before an operation. When it came to sharing my experience, I could definitely say that I had never heard of a knitter doing warm-up exercises before picking up the needles, and it suddenly seemed like the knitting world had forgotten a major part of their practice. Could our fancy knit moves be smoother if we made a conscious effort to warm up our precious apparatus?

The slow nature of knitting can cause us frustration and suggest the need to speed up. Fantasies of being able to present a garment for a special event, or knitting an impressive gift, are serious culprits in turning us into frantic knitters. Tight deadlines make it tempting to abuse the body, and just knit 'like mad' to the end. It is easy to ignore burning sensations in our fingers or aches in our shoulders and say 'One more row won't hurt' or 'I will rest tomorrow'.

Mindful knitters balance observation of thoughts with observation of our physical mechanics. At the end of each row, try to feel how you and your body have received the work. Some beginner knitters are baffled as to why they feel total exhaustion by the row's end. Are your fingers and needles at one with each other or are they being forced to work together? Treat yourself to a thorough pit stop, shaking out neglected parts of the body and easing overused joints and muscles with long, luxurious stretches.

YOGA & KNITTING

◆

Yoga, knitting and mindfulness are natural companions. Inhabiting our bodies in a mindful way ensures we avoid bad posture when knitting. After journeying with knitting and meditation, we can use yoga to bring our weight back to earth, unravelling the intricate moves our hands have performed for us.

During the early noughties' hand-knitting revival, I was rather embarrassed to be interviewed about the benefits of knitting, under a questionable newspaper headline 'Knitting is the New Yoga'. A recent student of yoga, I was opposed to the suggestion that one craft could replace the entire philosophy of an ancient practice in one broadsheet article. The strength of the revival was that knitters sensed the possibilities of self-improvement through their craft. Instead of replacing the study of yoga and meditation with knitting, crafters began to notice how ancient mindful practices can enable similar discoveries about the sublime, enlightened touch that an experienced craftsman can hold.

Yoga, knitting and mindfulness are natural companions

On investigating the term 'yoga' in more depth, I realized that there was some truth in the newspaper headline after all. The dictionary explains that the word 'yoga' derives from the Sanskrit root 'yuj' (pronounced 'yug'), meaning 'to unite' or 'join together'. By extension, this means to 'harness one's mental faculties to a purpose'. The knitting revival of the early noughties was very much about joining together. Forming knitting clubs to reclaim public places, we joined our mental faculties into finding exciting new communal purposes. Within ourselves, we used knitting to unite all our talents and moods. Discussing the meaning of yoga with my yoga teacher many years later, she pointed out that the word 'knit' has a similar meaning to the word yoga. Knitting and yoga are both about uniting; uniting people and interlocking elements. The word 'knit' has synonyms like combining, coming together, and blending. Most excitingly, knitting and yoga are similar forms of 'work'. Yoga guru B.K.S Iyengar, in translating the writings of the Bhagavad Gita, explains the term 'yoga':

'Work alone is your privilege, never the fruits thereof. Never let the fruits of action be your motive; and never cease to work. Work in the name of the Lord, abandoning selfish desires. Be not affected by success or failure. This equipoise is called Yoga.'

It is clear from these definitions that we could establish different types of work through mindful hand-knitting. Long investment of time for producing textiles becomes our privilege. Physical yoga poses help our bodies sustain these long stretches of industry. The different types of work we do within knitting can open up different parts of ourselves.

Why Do We Do It?

Motives for making are usually the desire for the object seen in our mind's eye. The excitement of imagining the object and then actually making something similar to your original vision is a phenomenal life experience. Our successes can be the overriding factor in our motivation for making the next thing. The more you get, the more you want! Completing projects is a great achievement in itself, as so many ideas never reach their conclusion. Through the celebration of finishing projects, it is easy to forget the gift of what we have learned along the way. The process of producing, from conception to completion, is the privilege that prompts you to make more. With this idea as your fundamental incentive, you cease to be affected by success, failure or loss of the piece. Failure can even be seen as a gift, as it gives you opportunity for experimentation and new, unexpected paths of making.

Much of the 'work' that we do in yoga and meditation is physically invisible, and the same could be said for many of the visions that knitting inspires. Having an idea is only one small part of the creative process and those ideas do not have to be realized. Enjoy images in your mind or leave designs as drawings on paper. This is still a completion of sorts.

Having an idea is only one small part of the creative process and those ideas do not have to be realized

EXERCISE

THE YOGIC WAY FOR A KNITTER'S TEA BREAK

✳

Mindful knitting does not require you to become a bendy yoga fanatic; poses can happen in simple ways around the home. The first step is to recognize your body's call for a tea break.

When you are ready, stand up carefully, using movements that feel good and allow you to take in a bigger breath. Shake out all your limbs and stretch, inhaling one big breath. Loosely wriggle your way to the kitchen or other place providing refreshment. Put the kettle on by using expressive or useful movements, such as standing on one leg and then the other, checking your balance on your redundant limbs. Waiting for the water to boil, use diagonal stretches across the kitchen to hunt down the teabags and relieve stiffness in the side muscles or shoulders. Playing a favourite tune can help these moves.

For beginner knitters, notice your improved co-ordination. Rotate your hips as you pour the tea, letting your spine ripple taller and taller as you wait for the tea to brew. Stand tall with your weight evenly distributed across your feet while you take your first sips and nibbles. Enjoy the sight of your refreshment and ask your body if it wants to do any more simple moves before it goes back to work. Given half the chance it will. Work like this for as long as you need. Finish your break by rotating your ankles and wrists for a few moments, then sit back down to commence the next row.

KEEPING THE SACRED KNITTING SPACE OPEN

Knitting is often abandoned for negative reasons. Misunderstood patterns, wrong stitch numbers, feline attacks or having to rush off somewhere are all gloomy interruptions. In worst cases, we never return. When finishing, let's ensure the needles remain open to our arrival. Harnessing problems positively makes restarting easier.

CONSIDER THE MANY THINGS HAPPENING while we are knitting. While cruising along the rows or rounds, our meditation might be beautifully focused, our breathing flowing through good posture and our interaction with the universe loved and understood. Yarn glides with ease through our fingers. At some moment today this practice will end. Right now the experience is beautiful and we will keep going. A sudden thought mindfully notes that our last sequence of pattern is over and it is time to revisit our instructions. We find our place. Our half-smile droops slightly as a frown creases our brow. We read the pattern again and again. It doesn't make sense. This is a bit like being woken up unexpectedly from a good sleep. We measure, we count, recount and remeasure. Something is wrong. We pause. It is suddenly blindingly obvious that our meditative flow has been intercepted by a stupid mistake. Meditation teaches us to accept all emotions as they rise up, which we do, as we listen to a whole new wave of irritated thoughts.

Peaceful work is challenged, for we have encountered a disruptive blunder, either of our own doing or somebody else's. 'Idiotic we must be, trying to be authentically mindful and not really understanding what we were actually doing!' or 'The pattern writer is surely to blame for not explaining coherently what they wanted us to do.' Or 'Perhaps we should be blaming the publisher for misprinting the instruction?'

Gifts in Disguise

Acknowledge these thoughts we can, but do we really want them to linger around unsolved until our next knitting encounter? Protecting the peace we have cultivated over the last rows, our first instinct might be to put the problem back in the bag, box up the piece and carry that away with us instead.

Trials and tribulations can be gifts in disguise. Technical hiccups, which prevent the plain sailing we enjoy in our knitting, are hurdles, specifically put there to teach us how to leap with confidence into problem-solving mode. It is a natural human condition to feel beaten, but it is also natural to be in control and to win. Like superheroes, the faintest whiff of a pattern malfunction should fill us with strength and a lust to get on top of the problem, coolly sifting through the pattern parts until we find a smooth route back to rhythmic knitting. Problems do not block you, they present an aperture for you to peer into and study. Bring the problem into the present and notice how alert and ready you are to crack the mess.

Complications highlight how much we are in control of our work. Some problems may not be problems at all, we just need to approach their confusion in a different way. Often we go over the same problem again and again and know in our hearts that we are not truly looking for the answer. Cloudy or disengaged heads find it hard to follow thoughts through in depth. Becoming more present in the face of the problem, we let the clues and ideas guide us, facilitating a passage for the mind to actually work out the problem.

Be a Miss Marple (or Hercule Poirot)

Abbreviations in knitting patterns can be so very small, and a mindful approach when reading them helps us see the clues in every bracket, dot and comma. Some patterns assume you know which part of the garment you are knitting and which direction you are knitting it in. Orientating yourself some- times requires you to have the lateral thinking of a great detective. Take out your mindful magnifying glass and take responsibility for problem-solving. We know from crime fiction that detectives are always summoning up great bouts of confidence and flashing their torches around in dark spooky corridors. Your knitting project belongs to you, it was started by you and it will be concluded by you. Let it happen.

If a problem with the pattern has led you to wind up your knitting until another day, finish with the anticipation of gleefully cracking a major case. Next time, through a well-lit, self-assured, forensic deconstruction of the scene, you will love to overthrow the turbulence, dare to solve the problem and remain in charge of your knitting. If you dropped a stitch twenty rows down, why not take a crochet hook and attempt to pick it up? Enrolling fellow detectives to talk through the problem with you enables you to share the gift of power from new knowledge. Whatever your approach, the causes of the trial cease to be important when the way you solved the problem becomes forever part of your experience.

The Process of Refinement

Solving problems in a knitting pattern that you are writing yourself can be equally rewarding. Tricky thoughts about mistakes are bound to arise: let these thoughts lead you to the right answers. Influences are everywhere to help you as you work. Catch them if you can.

The assumption that a designer should work from a fully formed concept can be taken with a pinch of salt. Some designers have the pattern fully prepared before they start, others allow for changes to happen. The commitment of time we make to our slow craft requires us to have clarity in our direction, but this does not mean we can't add sophistication to our ideas. If you need to change your mind and unravel your work, you have not wasted time, you are just 'refining an idea'. Unravel your work as many times as you like, because good design is always heavily polished. The more you polish your ideas, the more perfect your design will be. Let the work take as long as it needs. As the yogi says, it is the work that you possess. Let your journey be a long and joyful one.

CLOSING THE SACRED SPACE

Fondly regarding each knitted stitch as it drops down a row takes concentration. Yarn is looped through loops, as loops of thoughts are exhaled through your fingers. Reflect on your experience as you faithfully pack your knitting away, ready for next time.

LEAVE YOUR SACRED SPACE as mindfully as you entered it. Once you have decided to stop, take a moment with your breath and re-engage with the half-smile, if you have lost it along the way. Putting your knitting away is a great time for reflective practice. Thinking about the experience we have just had helps us to focus on the things that really matter, notice how we are and think about what we want. Reflective practice is the easiest thing to avoid as we are likely stopping our work because we are distracted; but closing the sacred space need only take a few special moments. Here are some thoughts to help you on your way.

Closure of the sacred space is specifically about caring for your work and acknowledging what you have learned. Do not shove your knitting in a bag that also holds your house keys, hairbrush or any other instigator of tangles. If it needs to go in that bag, pamper your work by wrapping it in tissue paper for effect and plastic for safety. Likewise, do not leave your work out for sticky fingers to admire, smokers to exhale over, cups of tea to be spilt on or for cats and mice to destroy.

Tales of Loss

Until your work is finished, it hosts the sacred space and therefore needs protecting. To avoid 'sacred space closure', pack your work away somewhere obvious so it doesn't disappear completely because you can't remember where you put it. This might sound daft, but it really can happen. I once lost two weeks' work when I was travelling in America, simply because I was enjoying the scenery so much and must have dropped it somewhere. Retracing my steps and racking my brain as to where my last stitch was made didn't help. My massive blue Shetland Spindrift dodecahedron on 4 x 3mm needles never came back, and I still imagine it lying on the sidewalk in Boulder, Colorado. My story isn't as bad as that of my friend Sue, who has eternally lost a near-completed navy blue cardigan in the comfort of her well-organized home.

Horror stories aside, let us finish our work. If you have time, rig up the ironing board and steam your work every time you finish your knitting session. More serious knitters might want to save this joy for blocking or pinning the pieces into exact shapes once casting off has happened; but casual steamers sigh, smiling, as the knitting looks less handmade and more like it has drifted down from heaven.

EXERCISE

WHAT'S UP?

✳

Paw your knits, wind up your balls of yarn and start to reflect on your recent experience. Reflective practice is a great way of developing your own patterns of creative thinking, and its benefits can also spill over into other parts of your life. Answer the following question in your notebook under the day's date: 'What happened when you were knitting today?'

Try to describe the experience as best you can. How far did you come with your work? Did you make any design decisions? Did you solve any problems? What went through your mind?

Once you have clarified what happened, reflect on your memories. How did you feel? How did you deal with the practice? What thoughts did you have? What have you learned from the experience?

Theorizing on your reflections, start to think deeper. How did the experience compare with your preconceived ideas? Was the result of your labours expected or unexpected? Do you know any formal theories that relate to your experience? What could you have done differently to change the outcome?

Your theorizing can then lead to experimental thoughts. What could you do to change the way you work? How could you find a different design path? What kind of behaviour might you try out? As you grasp an experimental thought, do not worry about giving it a cohesive description straight away; a hunch can take you a long way. As you research around your hunch, clarity will come. The more you reflect on your practice, the more you will find answers and lessons in the most unexpected places, including the depths of your own mind.

CHAPTER FOUR

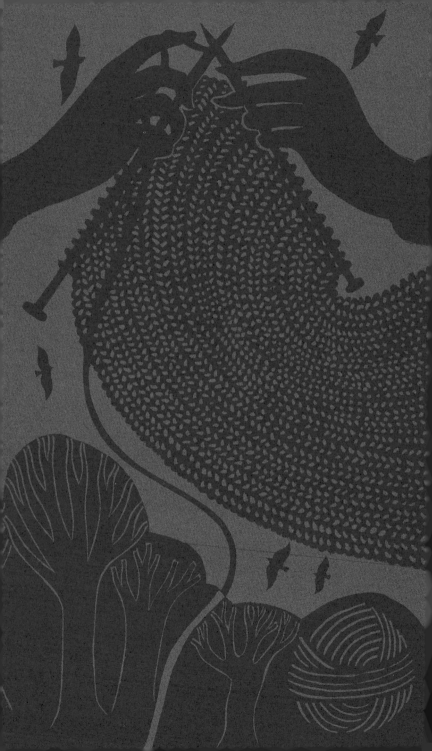

KNITTING CIRCLES & CRAFTIVISM

Craftivism is a word coined to describe the activities of a new generation of socially engaged crafters: Craft + Activism = Craftivism.

It's a great way to connect active creativity, social responsibility and mindfulness, and a safe and strong way to demonstrate your beliefs without shouting and waving banners. For generations, knitting circles have been unique social meetings where old and new friends are approachable for deep chat, simply because their work tells a story about their life. Crafty gangs form proactive, live, bubbling organisms, gassing with hopes and aspirations and often building platforms for cultural change.

CREATING MINDFUL CHANGE

◆

The funny thing about knitting circles is that however lawless you are in your creativity, you can't get into serious trouble. Or can you? Craftivism works best when you challenge people to question the way things are, and history proves that knitters are very good at that …

B YGONE TIMES HAVE OFTEN SEEN KNITTERS bringing their work out of their soft, domestic setting into brutal scenes of trouble. From the women who knitted liberty caps in between executions during the French Revolution to the women who knitted themselves into webs through anti-nuclear protests at Greenham Common in the 1980s, knitting often adds strength, harmony, colour and wit to protest and revolution.

My first knitting club had a very simple idea that we wanted knitting to be a socially acceptable pastime for young people to do in public places. The stares of fellow commuters while we innocently knitted on public transport had bugged us for years. Further astonishment from peers as we knitted during social gatherings in late-night clubs gave us the ammunition we needed to regenerate attitudes towards amateur craft and spare time. Why wasn't knitting normal? It was, after all, only a clever, practical and deeply enjoyable craft.

In order to prove our point, we needed to get in some sort of soft trouble, which would help generate sympathy for our cause. Our fortune came when we were asked to leave the

American Bar at the Savoy hotel in London for having too much of a good time. About twenty of us were dressed up to the nines, enjoying a few gin cocktails and teaching the hotel guests to knit. As the numbers of knitters grew, the waiter reached a point where he couldn't cope with the activity. To be fair, we were purchasing our drinks with vouchers found in a weekly newspaper; naughty but perfectly legal. Our eviction was exactly what we needed, as we wanted to subversively prove the power of communal knitting while apparently doing nothing wrong. Our story hit the tabloid newspapers the next day. People wrote to commiserate with us on our 'unfair dismissal', and from then on we started to notice flags waving for the public acceptance of knitting.

The Misses Marple & Carter

George Pollock's 1960s' film of Agatha Christie's detective Miss Marple, starring Margaret Rutherford, subtly summed up the complex naughtiness of knitting in a public place. Miss Marple is sitting in the public gallery of a court, silently knitting while patiently listening to proceedings. The judge turns to her and says, 'Miss Marple, either you stop knitting or I stop judging.'

The judge cannot concentrate on his work because the knitting is distracting him. I would suggest that he is put off his train of thought because, in his mind, the knitting is misplaced and should only be worked on in the home. By knitting through the long court session, Miss Marple is relaxed and able to concentrate more on the details of the proceedings than the judge is. Miss Marple is a great example of someone who governs herself by her conscience and not by the rules of others.

In the same decade, a maths teacher from our village, Miss Carter, was also requested to stop knitting in public. Miss Carter was an unusual character, and because her voice was so low she was the only lady in the village allowed to sing in the men's choir. She was an active member of the local parish council and made extra use of her time in the meetings by knitting red socks throughout. In the atmosphere of the times, this was considered inappropriate behaviour, eccentric and embarrassing. Miss Carter's socks were laughed at so much that her story eventually appeared in *Private Eye*, a popular national magazine that mocks current affairs.

Craft Aids Concentration

Today, Miss Marple and Miss Carter's economizing use of time might be considered quirky. My mother is a magistrate and often takes her tapestry to court for something to do during long waiting periods. She finds her work relieves stress and relaxes her mind before she goes back to court, where her thinking processes can flow and better justice is dispensed.

Miss Marple, Miss Carter and my mother all stuck up for their rights to work on a 'domestic craft' in a public place while being fully aware of complicated issues being discussed around them. In all three cases, the craft aids concentration. It should not be possible to get in trouble for knitting in public like this, but in heavily structured situations, it can happen. If you do get told off, you might be able to prove an injustice in an instant, or you might have stumbled on a thought-provoking situation where the function of knitting needs to be discussed. Fear of punishment is the punishment, so why not ditch the fear and see what happens. Liberating ourselves from fear of ridicule is a major step towards making public displays of crafted activism.

CRAFTIVISM

Working for good and making positive change is a primary motivation for creative people. Caring deeply about the world, creatives do not always want to be caught up in the noise or violence that fighting for justice can generate. Craftivism can be a soft, quiet protest, where producing thoughtful designs helps deliver a deep message.

THROUGHOUT HISTORY, craftivists have made the world a better place. Impoverished communities make textiles through good times and bad, supporting families who need extra care. A family's struggle through war, displacement of home, lack of medical care or accidents at work might be comforted by the generosity of a quilt or blanket made by friends. In the days before women had the vote, crafting was

The creation of things by hand leads
to a better understanding of democracy,
because it reminds us we have power.

BETSY GREER
AMERICAN WRITER WHO POPULARIZED THE TERM 'CRAFTIVISM'

another way of supporting the causes they cared about. Craftivist acts like these often become historical documents, leaving descriptive clues within the fabric about a community at a certain time.

A few years ago I was curating a daunting public craftivist project, and seeking inspiration I wrote to the former Bishop of Leicester, the Right Reverend Richard Rutt, who was a great knitter and expert on the history of knitting. The bishop kindly wrote back to me with many useful thoughts, but at the end of the letter he alerted me to a very interesting passage from a removed section of the Bible called the Apocrypha. Ecclesiasticus chapter 38 could be considered one of the earliest craftivist manifestos. The passage explains how the craftsman finds wisdom through labour and creates beauty despite the hard grind of his work. Without the craftsman making our homes beautiful, the city will not be comfortably inhabited. Without the city being inhabited, there is no need for judges or councils. Craft is the basis on which civilization is built, because unless the people are happy and comfortable in their surroundings, there is no need for the jobs that the rest of society might do. When the people are happy, there is less need for law, order and councils. Sadly, the chapter does not mention textiles, but the experiences of other craftsmen are all related to the work that we do.

Finding the Power of Democracy in Your Hands

Craftivist practice helps us question everything around us. Challenging established structures of thinking about craft itself can cause shifts in our actions. Even if you grew up in an open-minded, creative home, there is always more to discover about the origins of how we think. Sitting in a room full of diverse people who knit while seeing each other as equal is the first step. Our knitting gives us the peace to concentrate on and allow for other people's opinions while fine-tuning our own. Listening to the community and asking questions opens up our world. Craft has the power to take down walls we may have spent generations building. Once you stop labelling people as types and realize we are all just people with a craft gene in our DNA, the community voice becomes clearer and roles of the individual characters more important.

Craft has the power to take down walls we may have spent generations building

How to Start a
Craftivist Knitting Circle

———◆———

Gandhi's advice to 'be the change that you want to see in the world' could also be interpreted as an instruction to knit through the rebirth of your inner being, or to gather a tribe together and reclaim your ground. Cultural movements rarely start without a few like-minded people reflecting on a situation.

M Y FIRST KNITTING CLUB, called 'Cast Off', was formed after some hilarious conversations between a few artist friends. We were amused by fashionable society's assumption as to how we should spend our free time. After a long beer, stretched out by knitting a fair number of rows, we accidentally started a revolution. Our simple aim was to share our skills with responsive strangers, in a different place every time. At each event we would promote knitting as a healthy, fun and fashionable pastime for people of all ages. Our intention seems elementary now, as knitting in public has become so common, but in the year 2000 a socially engaged knitting club for young people was unheard of in the heart of the London art scene.

Causing offbeat sensations wherever we went, new groups of people chatted about the joy of making things. Knitting could be considered relevant in any situation, worldwide, and so it became. Creative sparks and positive action happened in unaccountable proportions, as people took their new skills back into their own communities. Our group quickly gathered press attention and new members with many voices directing its activity.

The Craftivist Qualities of Knitting

Craftivism as a genre can stretch across all different crafts. It doesn't matter how you make things, or what you make them out of, it is the idea and the interaction with the world that counts. Hand-knitting appealed to my friends and me as a craftivist medium firstly because of its portable, lightweight convenience, and secondly because strangers we met usually had an emotional attachment to knitting. New recruits typically remembered knitting a teddy bear's scarf as a child, or grew up loving someone who could magically knit anything. Re-teaching knitters unlocked portals to long-forgotten pasts. Reliving bygone cultures where knitting was respected, our new comrades were also surprised to recognize an incurable muscular itch on seeing someone knitting, where their fingers became riddled with jealousy and they simply had to join in. The physical and spiritual contagion of knitting makes it a powerful tool for craftivism.

Discovering the power in our hands, we began to experience nothing other than what we had altered ourselves. Taking ownership of our free time, new realities emerged alongside our completed knit projects and we all started to feel free.

EXERCISE

OCCUPATION OF KNITTING
AS AN OCCUPATION OF SPACE

✳

This exercise is about how to introduce knitting to a public space. We never know how much small-scale performances of knitting in public can inspire people to be creative. Inhabit a place for your mindful knitting practice. Knit there for as little as fifteen minutes and record your experiences. Here is how ...

Occupy yourself first.
Lisa Anne Auerbach
American textile artist best known for her knitting works

The word 'occupy' will take on many forms with this craftivist act. To begin with, we will occupy our hands with our craft, which in turn helps us occupy ourselves in the present moment. From then on, we can search for a lifeless place to occupy further. Take a picture of the lifeless place, print it and add it to your notebook. Make notes on how you managed to bring the place back to life.

If you are occupying controversial space, notice any self-imposed restrictions on where you allow yourself to be. Rid yourself of restrictions and knit as if there is no reason that you shouldn't.

When cynical onlookers enquire, half-smile and keep your answers in the moment. Comment on other goings-on, and enquire as to other people's activities. Express the joy of your occupation.

Should you be told to stop knitting, just stop; focus on your breath and continue to engage in the present.

At the end of the experience, reflect on the events of the day. How were you received? Analyse any restricting or uncomfortable feelings. Plan accordingly for tomorrow's knitting routine.

Collectively swimming in a soup of utopian dreams, the click of our needles became a call to arms, supporting the visions of us all.

Self-consciousness disappeared as we owned the moment and the space we were occupying. The stares of passers-by went unnoticed as we completed projects at rapid speed. Jokes were at the expense of any cynical audience spouting predictable knitting jokes, as we felt all the more proud of our mind-expanding lifestyle.

WHAT HAPPENS IN A KNITTING CIRCLE

Routine knitting circle gatherings are constantly in flux. Chapters come and go as projects start and finish. Competition smoulders as new skills are shared. Friendships unfold as seating plans adjust. Once your circle has a focused cause to knit for, it becomes a soft army, ready to gather wisdom and instigate positive social change.

YOUR CRAFTIVIST KNITTING CIRCLE should be a source of inspiration for legitimate dreamtime. Conversations with new friends can construct new situations in which to work, allowing you to experiment with new ways of expression. A knitting circle with a rich diversity of people can open up the traditional agreeableness of neighbourhood, with all its kooky characters, funny stories and unique meeting of minds. Ideally, an activist circle should introduce you to people you would otherwise never have the chance to meet. I have been delighted to knit with criminal lawyers, nuns, prison officers, archaeologists and all sorts of other professionals with whom I would never have had the chance to converse in depth had it not been for our shared love of knitting.

Textiles is an ancient, international language, making it a great catalyst for merging communities. Wherever we geographically originate from, textile makers form one nation, with a shared folklore and familiar conversation. Hush-hush opinions as to whether we could or would have made each other's creations is part of the emotional bond between makers. How many times have we looked at someone else's work and thought, 'I wonder how they did it?' or 'I wouldn't have done it like that!' or 'I wish I'd done that!'

We are all there to broaden each other's experience

However deep or fleeting our friendships are, we are all there to broaden each other's experience.

Finding a Comfortable Knitting Circle

Discovering a knitting circle with the right vibe for you can involve a long psychogeographical journey. Commitment to a few hours sharing your passions with strangers takes courage, but it can open up your world. Unfamiliar situations involving difficult gossip or unflattering critiques of your work are all part of this journey. Do not worry if you experience the wrong meeting for you. Treat it as a comedy occasion where you discovered the quirkiness of folk. However odd people might seem, in a circle where everyone's presence is of equal importance it should be possible to find something endearing or fascinating about each person.

Frustrating knitting club experiences can help you to become clearer about the kind of club you would like to see. What issues would you like to discuss? What items would you like to see other people making? When looking for action, be sure to wear your heart on your sleeve, being clear about what it is that you want.

My needs for a knitting circle change often, depending on the other things going on in my life. Having knitted in public for a long time I am blessed with knowing a lot of knitters, which gives me more chance to form a focused group when it is needed. Knitting circle cliques can be short-lived but highly valuable. Over recent months I have been invited to a very small circle of knitters who have all recently experienced the death of a loved one. We are all different ages, and we all deal with mourning in different ways. We don't always talk about death but the mutual support is present. As time goes by we may find that our need for each other fades, and all of us will understand that. Other transitory groups might be based around children, office politics or a local short-lived protest. Whatever the cause may be, ideas from these circles do not die, but mutate into new forms of get-up-and-go.

How to Form a Group Project

Relishing the here and now brings about fresh ideas. However wild the concept, tackle it straight away. If it doesn't work immediately, treat the idea as compost, letting it fester until it takes root. Immediacy in group projects is important as ideas are often not owned by anyone in particular. Unless you nail down the idea, it can fly off into the ether. Permit yourself to lead by example and invite your comrades to help.

Putting an idea through a creative process often uncovers a non-verbal communication. We have all been in a situation where it is easier to show someone what you mean rather than try to explain it. Let the itchy fingers of your fellow crafters continue the non-verbal conversation.

If your group project lacks product, or the others have got stuck on gossip, remember that the art of conversation could also be classed as a craft, and is greatly aided by knitting. Patiently pull together your ideas as you take notice, mindfully taking time to prepare answers. To thoughtfully make changes, you need to steer the conversation. Soak up the vibe of the community, listen to your heart and ask good questions. Navigate a way to share deep concepts. Individuals have many sides to them so look out for hidden depths. Learn to be a good host by bringing out the best in those around you.

Roles Within a Craftivist Group

The 'doing spectrum' is an imagined structure of a craftivist circle, where members perform different functions, with all the actions being of equal importance.

One end of the 'doing spectrum' sees the quiet, busy-fingered makers enjoying solace but wanting to provoke positive change and provide hope. These craftivists may be shy and feel isolated during debates, marches or demonstrations. The craft group gives a quiet person a supportive place to find a strong voice for their opinions. All activists have to strike while the iron is hot, fully engaged in the moment and putting their ideas into object form. Shedding the fear of knitting mistakes, the group can help the quiet knitter lose the fear of saying silly things in an unfamiliar social situation. The quiet maker creates the stability in the group, often giving much time and ingenuity as they nimbly work away in a corner.

At the other end of the spectrum are the makers who want to make direct vocal connection to the outside world, on behalf of other makers. These craftivists outreach whenever an opportunity arises, instigating projects, talking to the press, writing blog posts and collating the responses of the audience. Other roles might be the creatives who make sure the work can be made easily, and that all the group's work hangs together. Helping the work to be seen is as important as the making and these craftivists might nurture the project for a long time into the future. Vocal, organizing craftivists may lose time in the making process as their fingers are busy writing emails or installing exhibitions, but these skills are just as much a craft as material-based work. Mindful curation of group work requires perception of the community as a whole, empathy of all the individuals within it and a deep knowledge that the group is worth so much more than the sum of its parts.

Small Ripples, Giant Waves

Craftivists might notice how the voice of their group inspires other communities from different walks of life to pull together and make changes. Our very act of making can have far-reaching consequences, as American ethnic indie craft activist Faythe Levine explains when interviewed by Sabrina Gschwandtner in *American Craft* magazine in 2008. Faythe said,

> 'I believe the simple act of making something, anything, with your hands is a quiet political ripple in a world dominated with mass production … and people choosing to make something themselves will turn those small ripples into giant waves.'

When turning small ripples into giant waves, I like to think about those amazing friends we have who always get the party started. One person gets up on the dance floor, and then a second. When a dear friend gets up, and you love the song as much as they do, the urge to get up and dance with them can be immense. One knitter seeing another knitter in motion has an equally alluring pull. The muscle memory we feel on seeing our friends knit comes with a natural instinct to copy, and we become a knitting pack, as if once, thousands of years ago, we all formed one big loving opinionated textile machine.

The Comfort Circle

'The comfort circle' might take years to form, and when it does, it is very special. Loyal friends gather with knitting to check in on each other's lives, give momentum to projects and put inner worlds to rights. These circles are precious and usually closed to strangers. They might be held in private homes or cosy corners in pubs. Whether these circles are passive or activist, their priority is relaxation and well-being. Your presence in the circle helps you and everyone else tick. Your friends will laugh with you at mistakes, know which yarns you love and hate, give support with pattern problems and boost your delight at finishing a job. A comfort circle is not easy to find. Mine formed after years of public knitting and running a yarn shop. It is small and doesn't meet too often because we all live far apart, but when we do meet, I feel fulfilled and topped up with inspiration. Keeping in touch over the internet, I often feel the support of my circle and where possible take total pleasure in meeting for real.

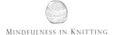

WELL-BEING IN COMMUNITY PROJECTS

Knitting is known to create a feeling of well-being. Facilitators of public knitting projects often struggle to cope with the emotional baggage people express when faced with making textiles in a relaxed atmosphere. The 'kindness' of textiles heals troubles over time, but it is sensible to prepare for their arrival.

WHETHER YOU ARRIVE AT A KNITTING CIRCLE with friends, or make an entrance on your own, the bravery of an individual to grace us with their presence should always be acknowledged. I sometimes find that new knitters have been summoning up the guts to join a circle for a while, and are relieved to find a friendly welcome. Braving bad weather or sluggish thoughts to get to a meeting could be a major achievement. A friendly welcome and good introduction helps a new member get started, enabling them to manoeuvre their way around the group.

A knitter could be joining your group as a means of escape from any number of problems.

The addictive quality of knitting can act as a wonderful replacement for repetitive afflictions such as irritating thoughts or other unproductive loops. The simple song of group chitter-chatter is the perfect prescription for someone who might not want to tell the group about their problems. Likewise, a grieving knitter is content just to muddle along, enjoying the company of creative people. Problems are not always immediately shared, and the knitter could be happy to take on a quiet role. People who do not overly interact with the group are still likely to be having a good time.

Acknowledge Progress

Smallest acts can become the greatest achievements, so it is important to notice them. We have all been comforted by our peers noticing our progress and achievements. Acknowledging progress brings a great sense of freedom and an urge to move on to the next thing. Part of the deal with achieving success and presenting it to a knitting circle is that you naturally swap skills with your friends. Helping the group master new tricks teaches you the art of teaching or, if you are on the receiving end, the art of learning. To teach and to learn are both empowering qualities.

People can be terrified to join a group project, for fear of wasting material. In planning a group project, make sure that badly made craft is as important as good. If a maker gives up through lack of comments, then they have lost the possibility of finding a resonating voice within. Fear of starting is similar to the fear of standing up and saying something. In holding back, we deny ourselves the opportunity to share something personal, or funny. Holding back stops other people understanding us or being inspired by our soul. A community is there to prove that fear is not a valid reason for holding back, and as an emotion could quite easily be swapped for excitement. Coach voices out gently. Even if it doesn't work the first time, it might the next.

CHAPTER FIVE

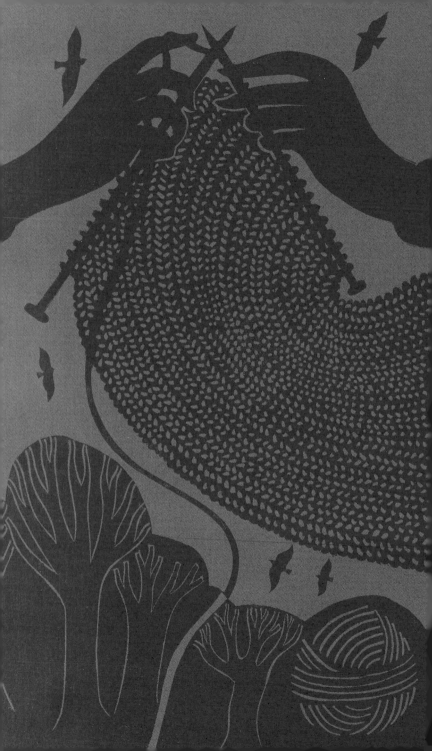

THE GIFT

*Writing this book is a gift for me. As I give
my thoughts to the page, new thoughts arrive, and
what I cherish most is the opportunity to share my
contemplations with fellow crafters who, over many
years, have generously discussed their own experiences.
I want to organize what I have heard and give a book
back to them all. Creative projects always contain gifts.
Mostly the gift is for ourselves, though hopefully also
appreciated by friends, and occasionally the greatest
gift is a mistake that we can learn from. The mindful
weighing of these values of gift leads us to a deeper
understanding of our reasons for making.*

THE VALUE OF OUR SKILLS

Knitting and mindfulness are gifts for life, at whatever age we learn. Years of practice are needed to fully appreciate the complex value system of the skills we have, but recognizing what we have received from our work empowers us to make more meaningful effort.

HAND-KNITTING IS NOT THE EASIEST career path to choose as the work is slow and the demand low. The problem, however, is a gift. I have been forced to look for new angles of profitable knitting-related work. Each project brings challenges of spiritual, material and financial evaluation. The questions 'What will I gain by making this?' and 'What will others gain by me doing this?' differ with every new career move or downtime knit project. When planning new work, others' judgement as to what knitting *is*, and what knitting *should be for*, complicates matters further when haggling in trade or collaborating on ideas. Back in our armchairs, our own judgement of what knitting is for evolves from year to year. I see 'the gift' of knitting as a fluid concept, ever maturing and inviting us to mindfully contemplate our ever deepening reasons for being, doing and accepting.

Gender Value in Knitting

History generally dictates that knitting should be classed as a female profession. Knitters know this is not the case, as men have always been expert knitters. The domestic image of the knitter often fails to highlight the hidden 10,000 hours that many knitters, male and female, have completed as they graduate into a master of their craft.

The way we can multitask with knitting makes it appear to others to be an 'easy' craft. Disguises of softness, kindness and homeliness all cover up the profound intellect knitting brings about. I have often been surprised to meet people who find it odd that knitting could be a profession at all.

We knitters are generative beings. Our work is initiated with a great compulsion to produce and create things, which we hope will be cherished. Other generative professions that could also be gendered as female are childcare, social work, nursing, teaching or the creation and care of culture. All of these roles are empowered with 'gift labour', that extra special something we wholeheartedly give in order to create a little magic. The energy we need to provide that magic is often unaccounted for and requires us to work well above the call of duty that other jobs require.

Work versus Labour

Every hand-knitter knows that the true cost of their handiwork soars way above that of the knitwear for sale on the high street. Contrary to some popular opinions, this does not make hand-knitting a lost cause. Rather than shying away from our confusing market value, we can mindfully focus on all our hidden profits, magically created through our labour.

I use the word 'labour' here because it describes something quite different from the concept of work. In finding the true value of our crafted pieces, it is worth noticing the difference in our feelings towards work and labour. A crafter may *work* late into the night, but wake up in the morning to see the fruits of their *labour*. Inspecting these fruits, we might experience an odd sense that it wasn't us who actually did the work. Unable to remember every stitch, we may only look back at the sense we had. Last night's labouring was connected to a deeper intention, which sets its own schedule and doesn't care about the time taken.

Mindful Inspiration in 'Doing'

Our intention to 'do work', or 'put the hours in', will largely be fuelled with willpower. Work tends to have a monetary value attached to it, or it comes with an expected reward at the end. Labour will always take place in its own time, and needs no self-discipline. If it is made with a heartfelt sincerity, it needs energy to materialize but tends to happen when we are in a relaxed state, possibly even losing track of time. Labour can even happen during a long bath time or serious lie-in. Geniuses throughout history have had eureka moments while procrastinating, and likewise, a knitter can find mindful inspiration through the dreamy repetition of their work.

Accepting our own sensibilities regarding labour and work prepares us for invitations to partake in the convoluted world of other people's economies. Knitters can easily become the victims of their own success. We can be offered commissions with an unfair gift economy or asked to sell works in an ignorant marketplace. If we become fully conscious of how we would like our work hours to be paid for or how we personally value our labour, we will protect the delight in our talents and the sacredness of our pastime.

COMMISSIONING & THE MARKETPLACE

When we make something fabulous, someone might enthusiastically ask, 'Will you make me one?' Before we answer 'Yes, I will', it would be wise to ask ourselves: 'Do I really want to?' or 'How mindful were the breaths I took to create Mark I, and will they deepen through making Mark II?'

PUTTING A PRICE ON SOMETHING you have designed with your heart and made with your head and hands is often a difficult, emotional decision, which has every right to change depending on who the buyer is. Balancing complex issues such as the price of materials, sentimentally over your labour, the hours engaged in work and your own urgency to sell is difficult. The price one person puts on your piece may never be able to cover the poignancy of finishing it. No one notices where you have picked up tiny stitches until your eyes hurt, or where you have ripped back hours of work to fix a mistake. For the craftsman, the obsession to get it right, and the respect for the material, means that we are likely to make huge backtracks at some point in our process and not count that as real making time. Sometimes we are ready to catalogue that emotional journey of making within our experience and let the physical object go. Other times we wish to keep the object as a guide to embarking on further creative experiences.

Repeating a piece because someone wants a copy for themselves takes you into a whole new value system of work. Newly experienced knitters will often mention second sock syndrome, a challenging trial where the excitement of proudly finishing a beautifully functional sock is quickly dampened by the frustrating fact that in order to feel the benefit of the sock, you have to knit another one. Second 'system' syndrome, experienced in other repeat knits, is heightened or lowered depending on your motives for knitting. The magic of labour can linger in repeated knitting if you have an emotional cause to knit for. Gratitude for the friendship of the commissioner, receiver of the gift or aim of the charity are common catalysts for work. Knitting as an exchange for something you could not afford in monetary terms is also a sound motive. The last and sadly rare reason for working as a knitter is to be paid a living wage, which in the age of mass production is unusual but not impossible.

Answering Requests for a Knitted Item

A typical challenge can be ignited when you proudly model your latest creation for the first time and your non-knitting friend takes such delight in your accomplishment that they instantaneously request a replica for themselves. Even if they are willing to pay you for the task, the legitimacy of this commission is not always clear at first. Unless your friendship is really close, the expectations of the commission for both you and your friend could very well be poles apart. If you, dear reader, ask me to knit you a yellow hat, and we do not understand each other's intimate language of colour, I may end up knitting you a hat that you can never wear due to my total miscomprehension of your idea of yellow! It is best to mindfully prepare simple, comfortable, yet thought-provoking questions and answers for challenging enquiries. Commissions can very easily pop up out of the blue and it is always best to be prepared.

The Amazing Knitting Grandma

Beware of the knitwear enthusiast who appears to understand the lengthy process of hand-knitting because they grew up with a much-loved grandma who would 'knit them anything'. Grandma was in the prime of her knitting career, highly skilled with time to devote to the ones she loved. Your friendship will never be able to replicate this love. The lifetime of dedication to her craft demonstrated by Amazing Knitting Grandma may sadly never have been fully appreciated. Your friend might see all knitters as possessing the same unconditional love that grandma bestowed upon anything she wanted, for no charge.

Counting the Hours

The slow nature of handmade textiles is not obvious to some people. The fluidity of our experienced movements annoyingly makes the craft look easy. Make sure your friends know how long it takes to make something. When they ask you how your life is, you might like to say 'I have just completed an eight-hour marathon on a sleeve and now I have to do the next one!' This is not only a more interesting news bulletin than the fact you have recently experienced a heavy cold, it will also prepare you for any future knit-related misunderstandings. If your friend moves on to asking you to knit them a pullover once you have finished this one, there is only a slim chance they have added up the hours. Championing the lengthy time our work takes is vital in a world where instant gratification buzzes all around.

Not all commissions are out to rob you. Fair and fruitful employment can be hugely rewarding and even life-changing. As maker and commissioner entwine in one garment, they both step out of their normal routine, making a stand against fast fashion and daring to discover the things they really want. As the maker helps the commissioner refine their taste, the commissioner can help the maker develop their practice by funding their studies and new ways of working. Commissioners and makers alike may have to learn to wait a long time for their dreams to become reality. Both parties care for each other throughout the waiting process and, as it draws to a close, together they marvel at the sense of wonder they have created.

Garments worth having are also garments worth waiting for, and even after the project is completed and time moves on, these garments evolve with us, and only get better.

WHEN IS A GIFT NOT A GIFT?

On a special occasion, someone who loves you dearly presents a gift. A hand-knitted beast of a garment emerges from the wrapping paper, screaming. Politely trying it on, you don't speak its language and can't tell it to be quiet or go away. You might think: 'Help! What do I do?'

THE LEGEND OF THE UNWANTED CHRISTMAS JUMPER is one that has been retold for several generations now. Popular culture has laughed at reindeer or Christmas pudding jumpers so much that it has now launched an ironic fashion for novelty knits in wintertime. Thankfully, this fashion saves the reputation of knitters who find knitting fun, having jolly visions of their loved ones modelling novel designs. Many a knitter has sped up their knitting towards a special family occasion, with the exhilarating anticipation of the gift's presentation adding momentum to the work. The love buzz of clothing for our dearest folk carries us through any dull second sleeve. As we imagine the inhabited garment igniting a party popper in celebration of the masterpiece, we glide through the blocking and stitching up with ease. With all this positive intention, how could the gift possibly go wrong?

Gifts as Weapons

Dr Joanne Turney, a lecturer in textile design and history, remembers the difficulty she had in accepting knitwear from her 'generous' grandmother: 'I wish she had made it more about me and less about her. Is it for the knitter or for the recipient?' So many knitters I have met have ghastly flashbacks to a time where a relation made them something brilliant, but because it wasn't fashionable they didn't appreciate it until years later. The speed at which fashions change when you are young makes it difficult for an elder to knit what you want at the right time.

The worst-case scenario happens when you receive an unwanted garment and feel like you have been attacked. The established idea that knitting is associated with love means that it can be used as a powerful tool. A seemingly gentle gift can be made with undercurrents of prickly emotions. A garment that has been made for someone you are not, but someone the knitter would like you to be, is particularly problematic. A perfectly acceptable, well-made gift can in fact be riddled with political preferences, class war and gender inclinations, as well as traditional or regional tastes.

Similarly, on entering a love affair, the sensual overload of deeply exploring a beautiful new friend triggers our creative impulses. Our emotions prompt what we think is a brilliant insight of colour and texture. All at once, struck with a charming vision, we wonder, 'How did this gorgeous creature live unclothed by Clever Me until now?'

Thank You, Darling, That's Lovely

Finding partners to sensitively buffer or accept your creative gifts isn't easy. However close our friends are, they don't always share our perceptions. I've knitted for a few lovers over the years, who for the most part settled into their garments. This was because we had a shared taste, although I didn't always get it right. The man I have happily settled down with, however, completely baffles me when it comes to taste. If I'm convinced that purple is the right colour, he will turn around and want green. I am lucky in that my perplexed partner will do his very best to understand and discuss my visions and, after much compromise on both sides, eventually wear my gifts with pride. It has taken a lot of creative restraint for me to get to this point, but I am content to trust that he wears my gifts out of choice and not out of guilt or obligation. Success aside, I do still occasionally miss the mark with my family at Christmas, who say 'Thank you, darling, that's lovely' and then end up returning the gift a few years later.

On presenting a garment, we can convince ourselves that the relationship is now sealed. But how is the sentiment returned? Saying 'I have made this for you so you must love me' is tricky. If the love is true, your intended should love you with or without your handicraft. To be fair, a knitted garment could make an insightful person fall in love with you, but in trusting this hope you will always be searching for the evidence in the wrong place. Our gifts should only ever be a clarification of what is true.

Mindful approaches to 'the gift' save us pain. Problems can be prevented with mindful conversations over sample swatches and pattern books and dates visiting yarn shops. Observing our loved one's reactions to colours and textures gives us a chance to escape our own opinions and investigate the deeply intimate viewpoint of someone else. Looking through someone else's eyes enables us to see things differently and makes our friendship with that person deeper. Not understanding their vision, this only gives a new subject for meditation. Let your loved one help you expand your ways of seeing.

The Red Cross Parcel

Mindful interactions aside, pity the poor prisoner of war whom my friend Celia's mother met at a party. As Celia's mother launched into a conversation about knitting, the man shook his head and told a horrific story about doing time in Siberia. For months this man and his friends patiently waited for rescue parcels from the Red Cross. They knew the parcels were meant to contain bars of chocolate, cigarettes and lots of other pleasures. Unfortunately, the postal service to Siberia took so long that by the time the parcels arrived, all the goodies had been stolen and all that was ever left was a miserable pair of hand-knitted socks. Socks for these men did not provide any buzz or make life any more enjoyable.

KNITTING AS A THRIFT ECONOMY

Thrifty people pop up in every culture. Whatever the style they pull together, these people are inventive, witty and wise. Thrifters want to get the most out of life, for themselves and for their loved ones. Thrifty crafters are never idle, forever extracting 'that little bit more' from life.

IN READING THIS BOOK, the likelihood is that you are a pretty thrifty person, wanting to get the most out of your knitting practice. Never wasting a minute, you want to think thoughts that are useful. The chances are that you are descended from many other crafty, mindful opportunists whose cups are always at least half full.

I come from a thrifty family, but I like to trace my roots of thrift back to the beginning of civilization. When I was a student I worked in an Iron Age village in Dorset, England. I'd like to think I'd make a good prehistoric woman. Decorating caves and hollows, I'd learn how progress happens in the moment, while contemplating the future. Catching gifts all day long, I'd make the most of sun for heat, rain for water and work for finding inspiration. As an Iron Age woman I could get frustrated and want to make better tools to build warmer houses and more productive farms. I know I get cross being cold, hungry and tired, so I'd start providing for tomorrow as well as for today, making hay while the sun shines. Some smart alec would probably come along and invent money soon, but I'm sure I'd carry on swapping my goods with friends, getting to know them better in the process. Whatever stage we are at, life is hard. Our thriftiness in fixing problems and providing for the future comes mentally and physically by never wasting the present moment.

The Practice of Thrift

Thrift is an ingenious, private economy, and judging by the amount of waste in the world today, it is not a natural instinct for everyone. Thrift requires us to swap our animalistic appetites for a more thoughtful approach to the present and future. Providing for the future requires us to mindfully connect the power of now with good aspirations. Like meditation, thrift must be developed through practice, with its competence and wisdom being handed down to us over many generations. Having a much tougher time than us, our ancestors found their thriftiness was ripe because the pressure to survive was on, and the mindset was practised every day. In the same way that meditation is easier the more you practise, so thriftiness pops up its clever head whenever we are stuck.

No great work was ever done without repeated efforts or failures. Finding the stamina to work through problems and produce something useful gives even the poorest people self-esteem, reputation and distinction. Our thriftiness in knitting might seem quite insignificant in comparison to the great thrift movements of the past, but the value of any thrifty knit is to keep the human quality of carefulness alive. Small thrifty gestures can inspire usefulness, humour and the genius that sets human beings apart from all other animals.

Thrift, Wild & Free

Am I making thrift sound nerdy and austere? There's nothing wrong with nerdy, and I do hate waste, but I see no reason why thrift can't be wild and free. Punk-rock fashion taught me to hunt out discarded materials and have fun making outrageous and bold fashion statements using materials that cost as little as possible. As a teenager I found punk very liberating to copy, as Vivienne Westwood encouraged her audience to emulate her designs. Letting nothing stand in your way of making a powerful image leads to creative visions about yarns in charity shops, or ripping up and knitting old sheets from attics and learning skills from dusty old library books.

The knitter's defiant power of thrift is likely to keep rising long after capitalism has peaked. Accounting for all the money we currently spend in our favourite yarn shops, we could easily conclude that knitting clothes by hand is not the money-saving activity it was during previous centuries. Ethically produced yarn for hand-knitting is expensive, as are the seductive books full of beautiful patterns. Most of the money we spend on ethically made, locally produced yarn is made up of the costs of reigniting a dying industry. If you add up the hours spent on your beautiful handmade garments, knitting appears to be an extravagant hobby for those people with 'time on their hands'. What is the point of spending up to twenty hours knitting a pair of adult socks, with yarn costing up to £10, when we can buy three pairs for £5 on the high street? Deep down, a knitter knows the definitive answer to this, simply through the experience of making. In clearly explaining this answer to a new generation, we also need to consciously recognize the traits of thrift on more profound levels.

The Mindfulness in Thrift

Mindfulness in its very essence is thrifty. It teaches us to find the highest value in every moment and make the most of all we do. Thriftiness requires us to think about the past and prepare for the future, but with our minds completely open to inspired thoughts of the present. Mindfully knitting, we recognize the labour of previous generations, who preserved this handicraft for us, giving us a heritage that keeps us warm and makes us look good.

The mindful thrift we find in knitting no longer competes with mass production. Our carefulness is about preserving our talents, connecting with nature, identifying with our ancestors and building a fruitful structure within which to experience enlightenment. As our mindful knitting moments become precious, time is no longer counted as money. Metaphysical investment in our knits turns them into priceless commodities, whether we are comfortable wearing them or not. As hand-knitted garments become old favourites, passed on from person to person, their 'cost per wear' becomes cheaper and cheaper as years go by.

BUT IS IT ART?

◆

The 'art versus craft' debate has been endlessly argued in knitting circles, with each side out-gifting the other with talent. Beautiful, functional and pleasurable things can have an emotional value equal to that of fine art. Creating things that touch people's emotions, engulfing them in loveliness, is a true triumph.

THE BOUNDARIES BETWEEN CRAFT AND ART have long been contested. Some people see them as important lines of clarity, simply because they want their practice to fit into a box. Obviously all knitters have a craft, but sometimes the things that we make need to be labelled as 'art'. Depending on the class or cultural background that you come from, both statuses are loaded with preconceptions, many of which might either not matter or be true.

Every knitter will have personal reasons for doing what they need to do. Many of the things I make are simply 'craft'. Sometimes I aim to make something useful, other times I think of a concept and produce a socially engaging object with no function and I have to call it 'art'. If I say I am an artist, I worry that people wonder how successful I am and if I'm famous, or how much my work is worth or do I get other people to do my work for me. If I say I am simply a knitter and I like craft, I sense people fantasizing that I failed all my exams at school and struggle to make a living.

Statement of Intent

Preconceptions of other people aside, it is comforting to know what you are happy to be labelled as before you get dragged into the art versus craft debate. How much do you value each of the two words, or do they have any relevance to your identity at all? Does falling into a category of art or craft change the value of your work at all? On which side of the fence are you most gifted: as an artist or a crafter? Is one of the labels the one you are and the other the one you would like to be?

Sometimes, recognizing the intention helps make the distinction. If the maker is trying to express something, perhaps that makes it art? The way we learned to make things also give us clues as to what we call ourselves. Long apprenticeships, learning every detail of making, tend to make us craftsmen. Forming our ideas into genius, honing an expressive talent, could mean we are an artist. Something wearable or usable tends to be labelled as craft, whereas something of beauty with no practical purpose might be called art.

Putting it in Context

Looking back through history sometimes helps us to value our work. The value of textiles has ebbed and flowed over the centuries. Tapestries, for instance, were ubiquitous in late medieval castles and churches. On a practical level, they kept out the draught, were decorative and could be easily rolled up and moved. The lengthy time and number of highly skilled people it took to make large-scale tapestries made them expensive, thus demonstrating the wealth and might of their owners. Oil painting gradually became more popular than tapestry because as the skills of the painter and paint-maker developed, so a disconnect between the production of the piece and the audience was made. In modern high art, it is often this disconnect that creates the prestige. Domestic crafts like tapestry and knitting are inherently popularist, because these days they can be made and enjoyed by all. Pondering on whether we get turned on by art and craft that is prestigious or popularist could help us place our own practice.

Having sat through many an 'art versus craft' debate, my own personal conclusion is that what I love about knitting is its versatility. Knitting is no longer about tea cosies and garments for all the family. Knitting can be yarn bombing, graffiti, protest, sculpture, painting, poetry or even a way of demonstrating science. The way people label themselves is equally interesting, but at the end of the day, we are all the same; one giant wave of knitters, engaging with the world in infinitely original ways.

Knitting can be yarn bombing, graffiti, protest, sculpture, painting, poetry or even a way of demonstrating science

THE GIFT OF COMMUNICATION

◆

As a universal language, textiles are common to all races, religions and classes. Travelling abroad, knitting in public not only enriches the journey but often grants a conversation without the language of words. Reciprocal trust and natural curiosity generated between crafters opens up travel experience.

WHEN TRAVELLING THROUGH UKRAINE along with my Russian-speaking brother, his friend was interested in my knitting and requested that I be introduced to his sister. The fabulously tall and stylish sister Natasha, with her heavy make-up, strawberry red hair and high-heeled black patent boots, had studied knitwear at a Russian fashion school. Natasha's mother prepared some tea while Natasha expressed a polite interest in my dowdy crochet squares and went on to show me her collections of homespun fashions. One knee-length blue and white floral cardigan particularly intrigued me. Knitted in a very fine, itchy, three-ply wool on about 2mm needles, it would have clearly been an enormous job for her to hand-produce. I wondered how she had had the patience to complete it, and showed my respect for her colourwork weaves on the wrong side.

To my astonishment, she said 'For you!' and made me try it on. My brother translated that she had made it as a final project at the fashion school, and she wanted me to take it home.

I will never know exactly how my Ukrainian sister felt about the cardigan. Beautiful though her knitwear was, she seemed a lot happier wearing her fake Italian labels. Did the textile culture in Ukraine have a tradition of giving away a special thing on greeting a foreign guest? Was it such a painful, slow-going project that she never wanted to see it again and here was her chance to send it as far away as possible?

A Cardigan Abroad

Back at home, as I watched the Ukrainian conflict unfold on the news, I was transported back to Natasha's elaborately decorated Former Soviet apartment and wondered if her wardrobe of fashion knitwear dreams was still safe and had excuses to be worn. Did Natasha send her elaborate cardigan to London with me for the pride of it being worn in a safe place? Should I try to send her a picture of it in various English nightclubs, or would she rather not know?

As the years pass by, I still consider it the most precious kind of souvenir – a ticket to view real life, and a priceless gift bathed in mystery and lost in translation.

Productive labour is the only capital that
enriches a people, and spreads national prosperity and
well-being. In all labour there is profit.

SOLOMON

CHAPTER SIX

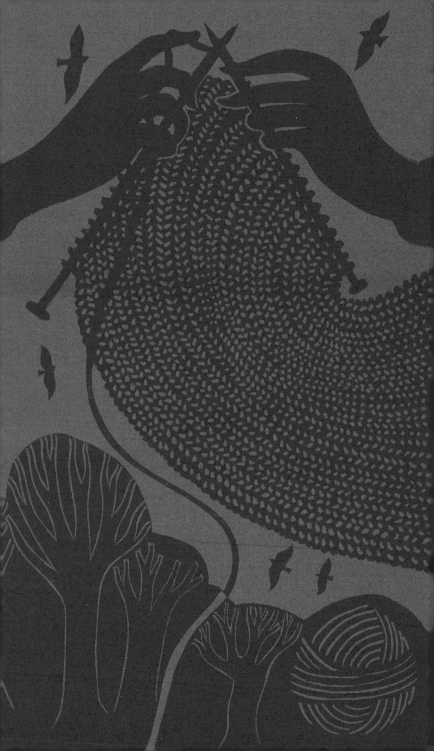

KNITTING &
SELF-DISCOVERY

*However peaceful we feel working lengthy projects,
the constant use of the same yarn does not always
guarantee a daily remedy for our colour-sensitive souls.
Perseverance on the long-term project requires a
different meditation from playing with the yarn and
knit stitches you lust after right now. Stopping doing
something, it doesn't mean you have rejected it; you
are having a look round another corner for something
new. This book can't promise to deliver you to a place
of enlightenment but it can direct you towards
unchartered territories. Let us now knit purely
as a voyage of self-discovery.*

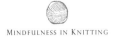

HOW TO CONNECT
MEDITATION WITH KNITTING

Throughout this book, we have explored techniques to increase mindfulness in our knitting practice. Sometimes knitting can become a meditation in itself, guiding us into our subconscious. Now we can start to experiment by letting our subconscious guide our knitting. Let the adventure commence.

TRADITIONAL MEDITATION LESSONS START by asking you to sit still, usually kneeling or cross-legged and with your eyes closed. From there, over a longish space of time, you concentrate on the pattern of your breathing. As your lungs fill up, you become conscious of air coming in, and as you exhale, you become conscious of air going out. As you breathe, you also become conscious of thoughts travelling in and out of your mind. As thoughts come, the mind simply acknowledges them without being identified with them, and the focus turns back to the breathing. To begin with, the thoughts come thick and fast, trying to remind you of your hectic life. As you become used to meditating, it becomes easier to follow the breath, and the mind quietens. A space opens for welcoming the thoughts we want.

If you haven't learned meditation before, it is worth joining a class or following a guided meditation on the internet. There are many types of meditation and it is important to find a guide you like the sound of. Be patient. Just as knitting took a long time to learn, so meditating takes practice. Combining the two techniques is an activity for lifelong learning. Never be afraid to fail. There are no rules. Once you have learned the process of meditation, you can start to notice the similarities between the in/out of breathing and the repetitive pattern of stitches. In joining a meditation class, you might also notice that it is decorated by a mandala or other decorative artwork.

Once we are introduced to meditation we can start preparing provisions for our knitting adventure. Intriguing yarns, varying needle sizes and stitch pattern books can be gathered into an allocated knitting meditation space. Here we will gather our ideas into a knitted mandala or shrine. Leaving superficial aspects of ourselves behind, we can dare to abandon established rules of knitting and knit in a more abstract way.

What is a Mandala?

In Indian religions, the mandala is a spiritual and ritual symbol, representing the universe metaphysically or symbolically. In the home, they can be used to establish a sacred space, aiding meditation. Creating a knitted mandala, either on your own or in a group with your friends, can provide the 'foundation stone' of your ever-expanding mindful knitting practice. Arranging curious sample pieces into a mandala helps us to enter a place where our hidden depths can continue to be

---

EXERCISE

THE VALUE OF YARN

✳

Start your meditation in stillness, holding a favourite ball of yarn in your hands. Close your eyes, or gaze into the yarn. Let the heat of your hands energize the ball of yarn. Focus on your breathing. Accept thoughts as they enter your mind, directing your focus back into the yarn. Once the rush of thoughts calms down, focus deeper on the ball of yarn. What is it about the yarn that you love so much? Where does this love come from?

---

explored. Allowing your knitting and your meditation to inform each other will also help you find more certainty in your creativity.

Knitting, meditation and the mandala can all be connected by counting. In knitting, we are often required to count our rows and stitches. In yoga and meditation, counting can help us focus on our breathing. The geometry of the mandala is founded with a perfect balance of numbers. Later we will look at numbers as a meditative aid in more detail.

Gathering Ideas for Meditation

Throughout this book I have discussed knitting as a lifelong structure for learning, a sacred space and a chance to connect with our planet, as well as ways to be an activist and ways to value what we do. Our variety of life experiences means we will contemplate these subjects in individual ways. Note down any strong connections you felt with these ideas, and save them for a future meditation.

Browsing in our favourite yarn shops, we are often arrested by stimulating selections of colours and textures, which sublimely reflect familiar aspects of our psyche. The itch to discover why these yarns turn us on can be so overwhelming that we guiltily lead ourselves to the checkout, emptying our

A Box of Unused Yarn

Eckhart Tolle begins his book *The Power of Now* with a tale about a beggar, who sat for thirty years on a box, asking for change. One day a passer-by says he has nothing to give but suggests that the beggar looks inside his box seat. Opening the box, he discovers it is full of gold. Eckhart Tolle goes on to say that in writing the book, he is the passer-by, with nothing to give us but the suggestion to look in our own boxes, which represent the inside of ourselves. I would like to illustrate Tolle's story by suggesting that most of us sit on boxes of unused yarn. Given the chance, I know that most of us would add even more unused yarn to this stash, such is our joy in hoarding colour. Boxed-up stashes represent beautiful inklings waiting to be explored.

wallets with complete lack of a provisional plan. We know there is good reason for this behaviour, but it is hard to justify it to ourselves, let alone to our friends. Let us legitimize these guilty pleasures, proving that impulse is only the start of an insightful journey. Accepting the intellectual interest in yarn cravings helps us unearth clues about our spiritual leanings. If every small piece leads to a new thought, then your time has been well spent.

LETTING MEDITATION GUIDE KNITTING

Letting meditation guide our knitting teaches us to challenge our expectations. As meditation teaches us how to overcome attachment to ideas, so it allows our knitting to change. Letting our intuition make colour and stitch changes leads to endless surprises, creating certainty in creativity.

CRAVINGS TO WORK WITH TEXTURES, patterns and shapes mirror the way we think. Meditation helps us to transform, discovering something new. Moving away from ourselves, and our established patterns of working, allows for plenty of surprises. When a new idea comes, repeat it like a mantra, refining its intention until it shifts of its own accord.

If you are shocked by what you made, try not to worry. Overcoming attachment to your original ideas is a vital part of creativity. If the yarn doesn't behave quite like you imagined, or you misunderstood the pattern, then let it be. Take the problem and fix it to your taste. Buddhism teaches us that attachment to anything is the greatest obstacle to spiritual development. Being stuck on something that won't move is a trap. Mistakes are the start of metamorphosis.

Metamorphosis is happening everywhere, all the time. Like seasons, real beauty is transient, always curious and rarely repeatable. Revel in revisiting something you made the night before, as if seeing it for the first time. Seeing 'things' in their infancy can trigger new ways of feeling. Accidents, blemishes or changes of heart lead to the unrecognized potential of an object. With no end to metamorphosis, we know that at some point we will simply halt and move on.

Knit Jamming

When you are jamming in music, you accept that there are no mistakes on the search for a good riff. Jamming with yarn and

In the creative state a man is taken out of himself,
He lets down as it were a bucket into his subconscious,
and draws up something which is normally beyond his
reach. He mixes this thing with his normal experiences
and out of the mixture he makes a work of art.

FROM 'ANONYMITY: AN ENQUIRY'
BY E. M. FORSTER 1879–1970, ENGLISH NOVELIST AND ESSAYIST

How to Make a Mandala

Traditional mandalas are constructed around big subjects, like eternity, purification, creationism, awareness or positive attitude towards others. They can be pictorial, decorative or both. The plan here is to knit yourself an adventure of self-discovery. If these deep subjects intimidate you then you can just have fun knitting something nice.

The basic form of a traditional mandala is a square with four gates, containing a circle with a central point. A mandala could also be constructed around a series of circles, squares and triangles. These shapes can overlap to form intricate decorations, as found in Islamic geometric patterns. Before you start, research the structures of traditional mandalas. There are many good books to choose from and lots of images on the internet. Mandalas are often balanced, rhythmical and mathematical.

In making your plan, rough out some basic school geometry shapes on a sheet of paper or a piece of material. Use a pair of compasses or a pencil on a piece of string attached to a pin at your centre point. Have fun measuring out perfect squares, equilateral triangles and circles. Once you have made a preliminary plan, accept that this is only a plan, and is allowed to change. The next stage is to consider what you would like to knit.

Are you craving a certain shape or colour at the moment? Your craving might be a series of shapes, or blend of colours or a more specific image. Cook up the fix you need by making a small-scale sample of whatever it is. Once a shape is made, repeat it, letting multiples bring more rhythm and power. Arrange shapes in the mandala structure and take a break.

Notice your relationship to your work while you are away. On your return, you may be conscious of what your work needs. If no ideas come, look at your work as if for the first time and be conscious of your reaction. Engage with love. No shape or colour is wrong, only looking for its right place.

Calculate patterns for new shapes to fit into the mandala structure. Use graph paper to help you calculate your shape sizes, letting each square represent one stitch and carefully noting your number of stitches per inch. Be aware of your shrewdness in conquering mathematics. As you knit, breathe and count, continue your meditation. Associations with numbers are deep-rooted and personal, leading to even more reflections.

Let Mandalas emerge with comforting cultural symbols. As your pattern evolves, accept that this work may have no beginning or end. Let us move on from the idea that creative projects are 'finished'. Our knitting remains in transit as our life unfolds. Mandala is an evolving image which we make to guide us through our contemplations. As we grow, the mandala can grow too, with over layering, cutting, patching, darning, framing. I wish you beautiful encounters on this brave journey.

needles teaches us a different technique of problem-solving. Essentially, our knit jamming could be called 'designing' but I'd like to think this is founded on a more sublime process than what we might learn in art school. Through the knit jam, we aim to see a 'helicopter view' of our practice. By following our instincts, we can grasp ideas that hover around but can't be captured unless we tune in to air traffic control.

MAGIC NUMBERS

Working with numbers when creating our mandala is a meditation in itself. Let the numbers count stitches and breath. Focusing on the nature of numbers brings a deeper reverence for the mathematical construction of all things. Through our knitted meditation with numbers, let's make sure that 'everything fits'.

ALL GOOD KNITTERS ARE COMPETENT mathematicians, whether their schoolteachers agree or not. Counting and recounting, increasing or decreasing evenly along the row, or asserting a decorative pattern over columns and lines are all proof of our harmonious management of numbers. Lifelong relationships with numbers teach us their familiar temperaments. We often develop differing feelings towards numbers, whether they be lucky or unlucky or mark a birthday or house number. In accepting these attitudes, we can also welcome the idea that numbers run to infinity – much like

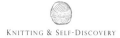
the action of knitting, with fabric growing longer and longer, numbers forming patterns, and the action of knitters the world over going on forever.

When designing our own knits, we often use a knit stitch bible, giving us many possibilities of patterns to use. These patterns ask us to cast on a multiple of stitches required to continue a pattern repeat. As these multiples are tallied by the invisible computer in our heads, we can let them take us on a worldly or supernatural ride.

Here is a brief study of characteristics of numbers, aimed to inspire contemplations while you knit. These ideas could enhance your existing knitting patterns, or they could be used as a principle for building new designs.

One

A plain knit stitch repeated over rows into garter stitch is the first number sequence we learn in knitting. An initial stitch is the seed from which everything grows. The very first stitch is simultaneously the point where we arrive in the discipline and the point where we depart into the freedom of creativity. Working fast or slow, our stitches are always a destination, landing us in the moment, and helping us delight in one fulfilled point in time.

As a first principle, the knit stitch is genius in its simplicity. New loops simply flick through old loops, one after another. To simplify the concept of knitting, we could say that one wiggly line passes through a previous wiggly line. A beginner may be challenged by separate stages of inserting a needle into the stitch, making a loop, pulling the loop through the stitch while letting the old stitch drop down a row. As the knitter streamlines their understanding of the wiggly line, they start to see the making of a knit stitch as one pure and simple idea, perfect in its completeness. As the understanding of a stitch's behaviour deepens, the knitter can develop a language of endless loopy manipulations, all derived from one simple stitch. The more stitches we master, the more we can welcome knitting as one unified, wholesome concept.

A knit stitch is one pure and simple idea

Two

Introducing the purl stitch to its opposite, the knit stitch, we see two stitches combine to form an entire world of pattern and texture. The knit stitch, made with the yarn and needle directed away from us, and the purl, made with the yarn and needle moving towards us, work as a duo to compose a bottomless collection of textures, patterns, drapes and stretches of textile.

Knits and purls working together can inspire us to think about the notion of duality. Essentially, the knit and purl stitch are the same thing, but they face in opposite directions. Unravelling a 1 × 1 rib, we see how all the stitches can be seen as knits or purls, depending on which way round we look at them. Another duality can be seen when decreasing a raglan sleeve edge: we treasure the neatly reflecting decreases of k2tog on one side and sl1, k1, psso on the other. Wherever twos occur in knitting, let them inspire different thinking about duality in your life, in one of the following ways.

The number two is essential as a basis for comparison. Once we recognize whether a stitch is a knit or purl, we become fluent knitters. In the rest of our lives, comparisons of this and that become the method by which our minds know things. Let the front/back quality of knits and purls help us consider the beauty of all opposites. Odd and even, positive-negative polarized charges, shape and shadow, limited or unlimited, right-left, up-down, male or female, resting or moving, straight or curved, sun or moon, day or night, and – our closest aid to meditation – the consistent in and out of breathing. Considering both sides of situations in your life, sometimes it is healthy to have differing opinions or mixed feelings. As knitting patterns help us to see opposites as balance, allow any duality in your thought to create a harmonious pattern, just like the complex yet simple fabric being made between your left and right needles.

Three

Three is the first odd prime number. Threes happen often in knitting, being a short sequence for the threads to travel across in intarsia, three stitches to think about (yo, k2tog), or three stitches over which to work a decrease on a raglan edge. As we work these, we can consider our wider relationship with number three.

The three stages of time in process, beginning, middle and end, possibly provide the deepest meditation on the number three for a knitter. The designed idea, the energetic work and the respectful conclusion and use of a knitted piece all help the knitter relate to completed life cycles. As the tree bridges heaven and earth, taking light from the sky and water from the earth, so the knitter bridges the heavenly design ideas of knitting with the making of a useful, earthly object from nature's raw materials.

On finishing our knitted masterpieces and setting them free to be used, we can relate to the Hindu holy trinity of Brahma the creator, Vishnu the preserver and Shiva the destroyer, all working together as one. These three appear throughout nature in principle and form. The knitter plays these three parts, envisioning the garment, making it wearable and accepting the destruction of their work by darning or re-knitting over time.

Giving thanks for the work we have made, we can meditate on three stages of time; past, present and future. Our skills are inherited from the past, proved in the present and preserved for the future. Fashion is also from the past, present and future, working neither fast or slow but all happening in the moment.

Four

A common 2×2 cable, 2×2 rib or textured brick stitch all work over four stitches. Comfortable number four is easy to count, forming the 4×4 rhythm of a punk-rock anthem or fourths in major or minor chords. As we knit in fours, we feel our connection with knitters in the far four corners of the Earth, connected by four winds and a psychological mixture of the ancient four humours.

Knitters very often knit with the four seasons in mind; anticipating the coming of the summer or winter solstice and the spring or autumn equinox, our knitting is often fuelled with the memories of seasons past and the anticipation of times ahead. As we design our project for seasons ahead, we are likely to pass a memory of the four classical elements of fire, earth, air and water. Like four old friends, the existence and properties of these four elements are known directly to us in a primeval perception. As seasons change, so our sensory experience of these elements changes.

Born under the zodiac sign of Aries, I am a fire sign. I am not an expert on astrology but I do know that my love of knitting is deeply connected to inward and outward natures of heat. I love the inner cosiness generated by my body under layers of wool, sitting by an open fire in winter. I equally love the freeing protection that wool provides while I dance around a bonfire on a midsummer's night, protected from the fire's scorching by a lightweight cardigan. Experiences of the other elements, such as homely earth, light and breezy air and tidal surges of flowing water, appear in my knitting practice in unforeseen ways, which might be quite different for you.

Five

Born with five fingers on two waving hands, our sophisticated digits form the dextrous machine with which we learn to knit. As we become more fluent and experienced in designing projects, we become wise to the fifth classical element, Aether (Greek) or quintessence (Latin). In classical times, the heavenly fifth element was thought to work with the four worldly elements of fire, earth, air and water, the fifth element being that extra special something needed for creation to occur, and for immortality to be achieved.

The fifth element has none of the qualities of terrestrial elements. Classical scholars understood it as neither hot nor cold, wet nor dry, and nor could it actually be found. Alchemists of the Middle Ages thought, hilariously, that the fifth element could be found by distilling alcohol, but all along experienced knitters have known where to find it! The magic of the Aether appears as a project comes to fruition. As pieces of knitting are released from the needles, pressed with a steam iron, stitched together and worn for the first time, there is a feeling that we did not make this genius thing completely by ourselves. A great, sublime element has been at play, helping us turn yarn into something truly special.

Six

Knitting in sixes is great for focusing on where you are in the world, and how you will knit for another human being occupying the same planet. The six coordinates of global positioning – north, south, east, west, up and down – can help you draw a line between you and someone else, anywhere in the world. Perhaps you need to connect with an old friend or long-lost relation. In theory, a person in your mind's eye is only six degrees separated from you even though they live on any one of six continents or across any of the six oceans. Your extra perception or sixth sense can help you design appropriate knitted presents or prayers for this person.

As we knit in sixes, we can focus on its perfection, with all its parts adding up or multiplying into itself ($3 \times 2 \times 1 = 6$ and $3 + 2 + 1 = 6$).

Just as busy bees arrange their honey into honeycomb hexagons, so we can fill our six directions of surroundings with the sweetest of intentions.

Seven

Vikings counted sheep in groups of seven because seven is the highest number of items that can be cognitively processed as one single set. Often known as the magic number, seven seems to have been involved in constructing our universe for us. Perhaps Buddha walked the seven steps at his birth just as the Christian God performed creation over that seven-day week? Avoiding the seven deadly sins, we could explore the seven skies of Islam, the seven wonders of the world, or even count the seven pillars of the house of wisdom. A seven-year itch in a relationship can be troublesome but it reminds us of the Druids' seven-year marriages and their renewal of vows. If these ideas are offering too much cosmic travel for one mindfulness session, why not simply give thanks for the seven colours of the rainbow, work seven rows of your knitting and find the seventh heaven it provides.

Eight

Love them or hate them, the eight-legged spider is our friend as she spins the most sophisticated webs, with far less tangles than we get ourselves in. Knitters' affiliation with spiders started long ago when Roman weaver Arachne challenged the goddess of wisdom and crafts, Athena, to a competition over who could make the finest cloth. There are several versions of this story; this is Ovid's version from *Metamorphoses*.

Arachne, having woven from an early age, was a fantastic weaver, but boasted that her skill was greater than that of Athena and refused to acknowledge that her skill came, in part at least, from the goddess. Athena, having been insulted, challenged Arachne to a weaving contest. Dressed as an old lady, she approached arrogant Arachne with words of warning: 'You can never compare to any of the gods. Plead for forgiveness and Athena might spare your soul.'

'Ha! I only speak the truth and if Athena thinks otherwise then let her come down and challenge me herself,' Arachne replied. Removing her disguise, beautiful Athena appeared in a sparkling white chiton, and the two began to weave. Athena's weaving represented four contests between mortals and the gods, where the gods punished mortals for setting themselves as equals of the gods. Arachne's weaving depicted ways that the gods had misled and abused mortals. She was particularly cross with Zeus for tricking and seducing women. When Athena saw that Arachne had insulted the gods, with weaving far more beautiful than her own, she was infuriated. Ripping Arachne's work to shreds in a rage, she turned her into a spider and cursed her and her descendants to weave forever.

As knitting appeared later than weave, I think that it is safe to say that we too are descended from Arachne, as we are destined to need cloth for all time.

Nine

Knitting on cloud nine must be the most blissful of all the meditations, especially in the company of a purring cat with nine lives! Safe in the knowledge that you made a stitch in time, saving nine, means you are well on the way to avoiding the nine circles of hell, which only beckon wayward and lazy people. Human pregnancy gives you a whole nine months of forward-looking knitting, or you can meditate with the Beatles, on a wild revolution number nine.

Ten

Born in the 1970s, I am a child of the decimal and love the neatness of stacking up in groups of ten. My mother, however, is an imperial lady and much prefers the structure of twelves. If decimal provides a comfortable structure for you, enjoy counting in tens, letting your inner calculator work with you.

Bored of accounting, you could switch to clouds, there being ten different types, which when learned could gently waft through your imagination.

A Greater Understanding

As we hurtle towards the end of this chapter and also the end of this book, I expect our study of mindful knitting to expand in many unique directions. Despite an entire book spent in the contemplation of knitting, our study of patterns and thought has only just begun. The ancient arts of textiles, mathematics and mindfulness all have worked together for thousands of years and we are just one minute generation, re-evaluating the best way to work.

Whether we want to knit complex masterpieces or plain scarves, our practice plays a vital part in the great awareness of humanity. In a time where humanity might appear to us to have lost its awareness, everything that we think, say or do has the power to send a ripple of enchanting positivity into our community. Every ripple sent inspires someone near us to have a go at something good.

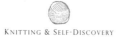
Whatever we knit from now on, we will no longer regard it merely as decoration or a layer to protect us from the weather. Like the structure of Islamic patterns, our handmade decorations and public displays of craft are also there to lead the viewer to a greater understanding of an underlying reality. Mindful knitting can help us discover how the world works. Adding beautiful patterns to functional things, we see decoration as a transformation. We start to know how transformation works. Allowing beautiful patterns into our thinking also creates transformation. Let the transformation bring more light into our lives. Let the lessons we learn open windows onto the infinite. Let us clothe ourselves twice.

INDEX

INDEX

...WLEDGEMENTS

◆

...de to the workers, exhibitors, customers ...t Prick Your Finger for the conversation, ...ners' at Art Workers' Guild for widening that ...tion, to my yoga and meditation teacher Sallyanne ...d for letting the conversation settle, and to my mother, ...other and husband for providing the peace within which to write. Thanks also go to the patient editors at Leaping Hare Press for their mindful advice and encouragement. This book is dedicated to my father and son, my father passing away as my son and this book were in utero.